GLUTEN-FREE SOURDOUGH BREAD MACHINE COOKBOOK

A Beginner's Step-By-Step Guide To Baking Homemade Irresistible No-Wheat Loaves With Your Bread Maker

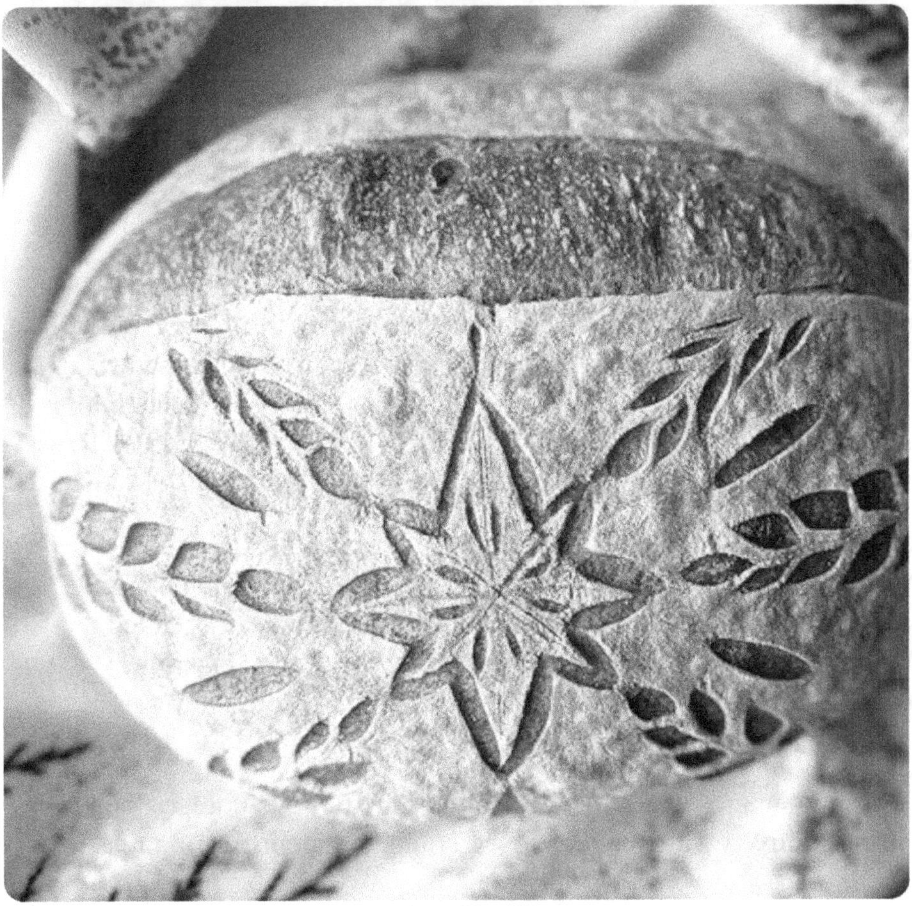

Beatrice R. Kramer

Copyright © [2024]

Designed and created by Beatrice R. Kramer

For permission, contact [beatricekramerhelp@gmail.com]

Beatrice R. Kramer lovingly prepared and tested the recipes in this book. All recipes have been updated and developed with everyone in mind, inspiring people to discover the joy of baking and creating tasty slices of bread.

GET OTHERBOOKS FROM THIS AUTHOR BY SCANNING THE CODE BELOW

INTRODUCTION

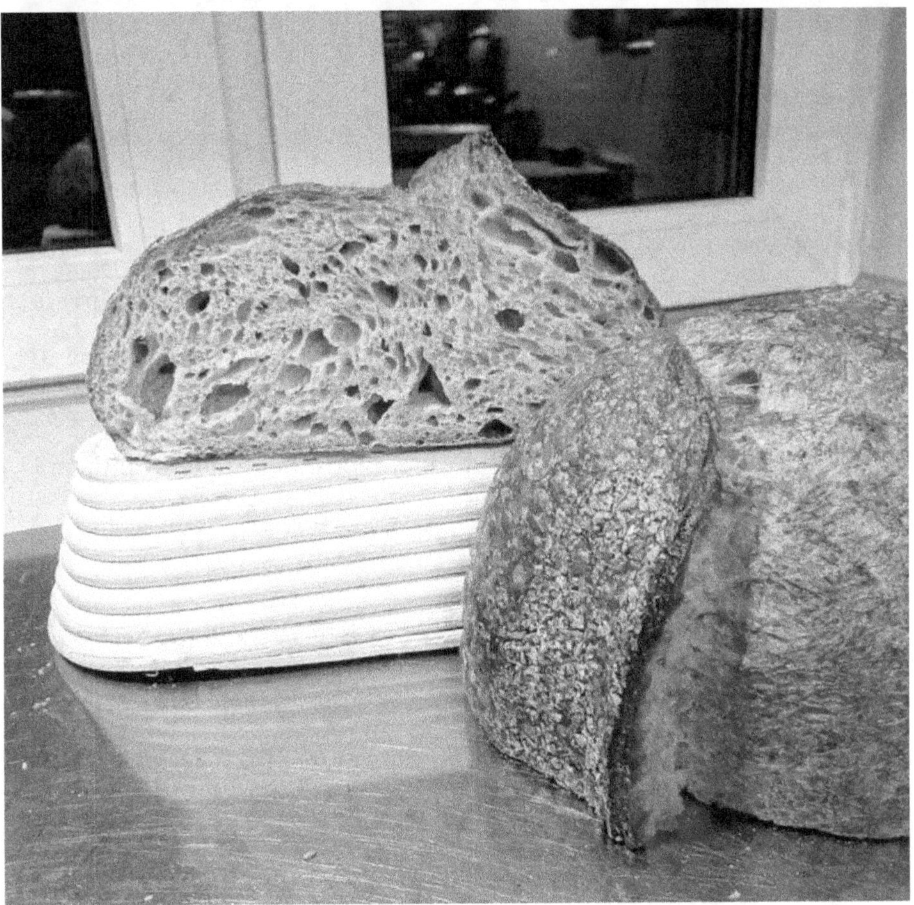

Welcome to a world where the warm, comforting aroma of freshly baked sourdough bread doesn't have to be a distant dream for those on a gluten-free diet.

The "Gluten-Free Sourdough Bread Machine Cookbook" is your guide to mastering the art of baking delicious, gluten-free sourdough bread with ease and joy.

Imagine Sophia, a mother of two, who recently discovered her gluten intolerance. Like many, she thought her days of enjoying homemade bread were over. The store-bought gluten-free options were either too dense or lacked flavor, and her attempts at homemade bread were frustrating – loaves that didn't rise, or worse, crumbled to pieces. Sophia's story is not unique. It echoes the challenges faced by thousands who, due to health or dietary choices, have said a reluctant goodbye to gluten.

But why should anyone miss out on the joy of sourdough baking? Why should 'gluten-free' mean 'free from taste' or 'free from the joy of baking'? These are the questions that inspired the creation of this book.

This guide is not just a collection of recipes; it's a journey into the heart of gluten-free sourdough baking. Each page is packed with information, tips, and step-by-step processes designed to take you from a curious novice to a confident baker. You'll learn the secrets of preparing the perfect gluten-free sourdough starter – the soul of every sourdough loaf. You'll discover how to choose the right gluten-free flours and how to make your bread machine your best ally in this adventure.

We'll tackle common challenges head-on. Does your bread not rise as you hoped? We have the solutions. Crumbly texture? We'll show you how to achieve that perfect, tender crumb. Each recipe has been crafted to ensure success, bringing you the same joy of baking that Sophia discovered.

From classic loaves to innovative creations, every recipe in this book is a step towards demystifying the world of gluten-free sourdough baking. Whether you're craving a rustic loaf, a sweet and savory treat, or something unique for a special occasion, this book has it all.

Most importantly, this cookbook is about celebrating the joy of baking and the satisfaction of enjoying something made with your own hands. It's about not letting dietary restrictions limit your culinary adventures. With this book, gluten-free sourdough bread is not just possible; it's delicious, rewarding, and fun.

So, preheat your bread machine, and let's embark on this gluten-free sourdough journey together

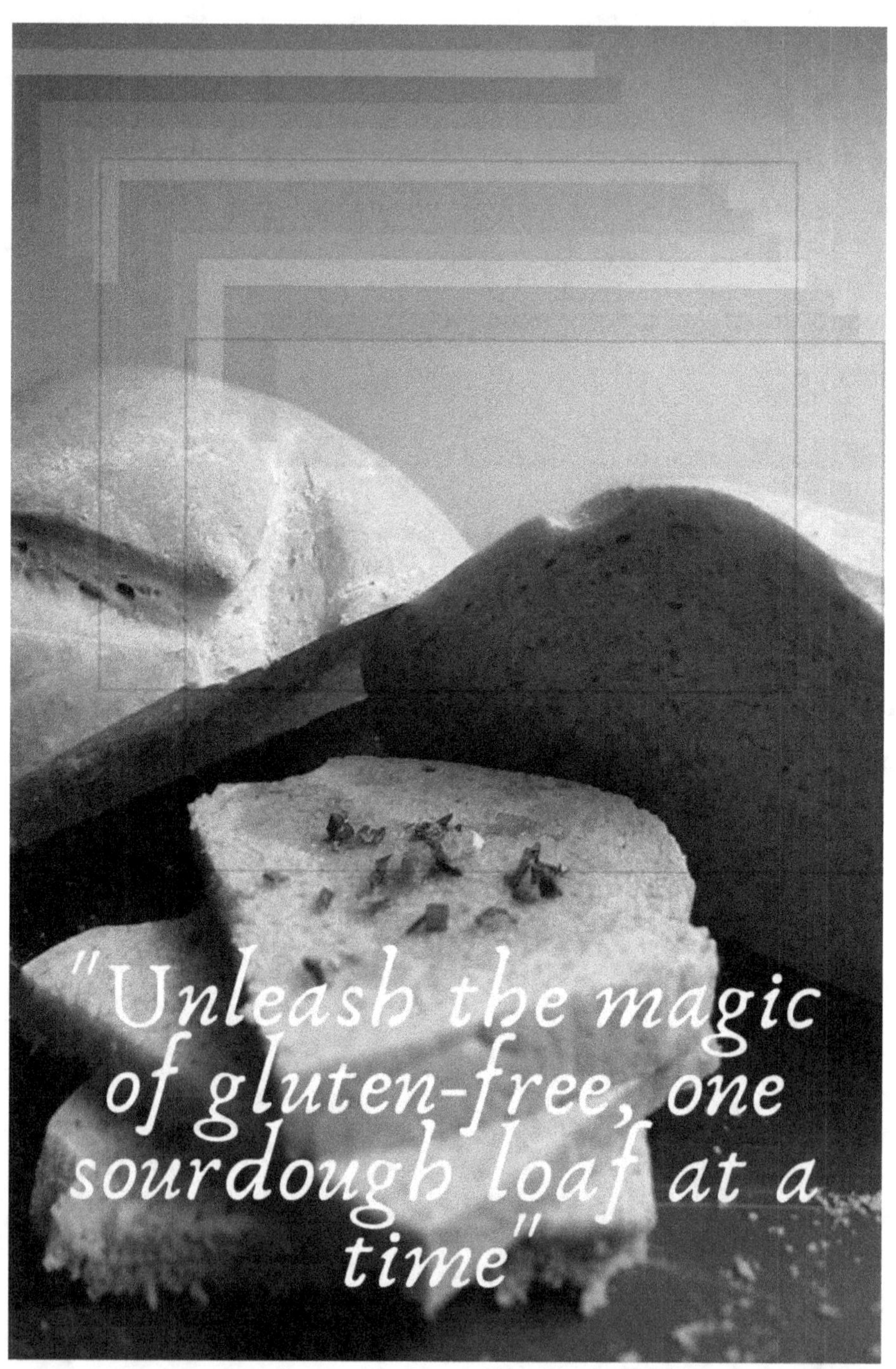
"Unleash the magic of gluten-free, one sourdough loaf at a time"

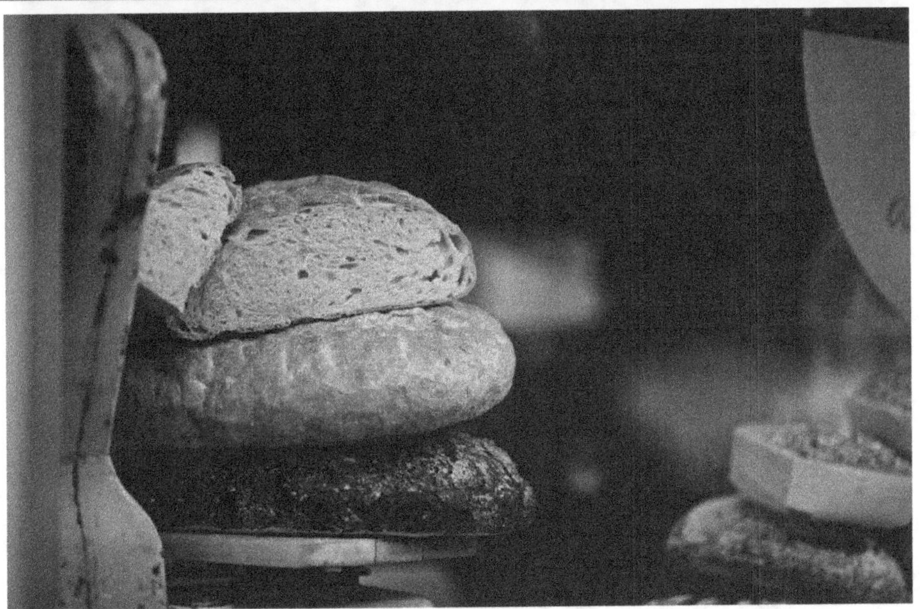

CHAPTER 1

Introducing to Gluten-Free Sourdough Baking

Choosing the gluten-free sourdough baking world, a joyful and nutritious adventure that guarantees both deliciousness and health. In this chapter, you will find the necessary information to create gluten-free sourdough bread in a bread machine.

What Does Gluten-Free Mean?

Firstly, let's demystify 'gluten-free'. Gluten is a protein found in wheat, barley, and rye. For individuals with celiac disease, gluten intolerance, or those who simply choose a gluten-free lifestyle, consuming gluten can lead to various health issues. Gluten-free baking, therefore, means preparing baked goods without any of these gluten-containing grains. Instead, we use alternative flours like rice, almond, or buckwheat flour, which are not only safe but also add unique flavors and textures to our bread.

The Benefits of Sourdough

Sourdough bread, with its signature tangy flavor, is not only delicious but also beneficial for your health, especially when it's gluten-free. The long fermentation process of sourdough can make it easier to digest and can help in nutrient absorption. It often has a lower glycemic index, which is advantageous for blood sugar control. Sourdough fermentation also reduces the presence of phytates, which can inhibit the absorption of minerals.

Using Your Bread Machine Effectively

Now, let's talk about your bread machine, an invaluable ally in this gluten-free sourdough adventure. Bread machines are not just convenient; they provide a controlled environment for bread baking, which is crucial for gluten-free breads. They take care of the mixing, kneading, rising, and baking, ensuring consistent results.

> Know Your Machine: Familiarize yourself with your bread machine's settings. Gluten-free bread usually requires a different setting than regular bread due to its unique kneading and rising requirements.

> Temperature Matters: Ingredients should be at room temperature unless otherwise specified. This ensures better yeast activation and dough consistency.

> Order of Ingredients: Generally, liquids go in first, followed by dry ingredients, and yeast last. This order prevents the yeast from activating too soon.

> Scrape the Sides: Occasionally, you might need to scrape down the sides of the bread pan during the initial mixing to ensure all ingredients are well incorporated.

> Monitor the Dough: Gluten-free dough should resemble a thick batter. If it's too dry or too wet, don't hesitate to adjust by adding a little water or flour.

Say along!

"Every time I bake a gluten-free sourdough loaf, I'm creating a delicious masterpiece, proving that my culinary skills can bring joy and healthiness to every bite. I am talented, capable, and transforming the world of baking. I am a master of transformation, skillfully crafting gluten-free sourdough bread that nourishes the body and delights the soul."

The Essentials of Gluten-Free Baking

Being a gluten-free sourdough baker requires familiarizing yourself with some essential ingredients and tools. This chapter will guide you through everything you need to start baking delicious, wheat-free sourdough bread in your bread machine.

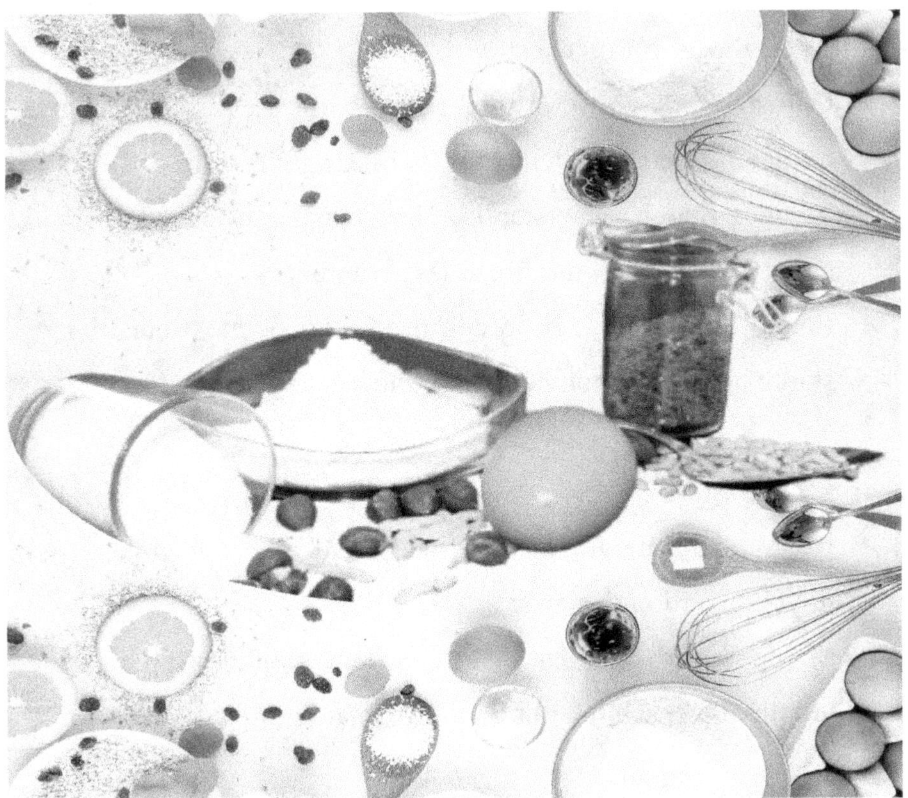

Flour Alternatives for Gluten-Free Sourdough

- ➢ Rice Flour: A staple in gluten-free baking, rice flour is versatile and light. It's an excellent base for your flour blends.

- ➢ Almond Flour: Rich in flavor and nutrients, almond flour adds moistness and a nutty taste to your bread.

- ➢ Buckwheat Flour: Despite its name, buckwheat is entirely gluten-free and imparts an earthy, rich flavor.

- ➢ Sorghum Flour: High in protein and fiber, sorghum flour lends a mild, sweet flavor to your sourdough.

Essential Grains and Starches

- ➢ Cornstarch: A go-to for thickening, cornstarch is also integral to gluten-free flour blends for its fine, light texture.

- ➢ Tapioca Starch: This starch is key for adding chewiness and structure, making your bread less crumbly.

- ➢ Potato Starch: Not to be confused with potato flour, potato starch helps add moisture and lightness to your bread.

Natural Sweeteners

- ➢ Honey: Adds natural sweetness and can help to feed the yeast in your sourdough starter.

- ➢ Maple Syrup: A great vegan option, maple syrup lends a unique flavor while aiding in fermentation.

> Agave Nectar: Another vegan-friendly sweetener, agave is perfect for adding sweetness without overpowering flavors.

Vital Bread Machine Equipment

> Bread Machine with Gluten-Free Setting: Essential for consistent results, as gluten-free bread requires different kneading and rising times.

> Paddles: Ensure your bread machine comes with paddles suitable for mixing heavier gluten-free doughs.

> Measuring Cups and Spoons: Accuracy is key in baking, so a good set of measuring tools is essential.

> Digital Scale: For precise measurement of ingredients, a digital scale is a valuable tool.

> Thermometer: To check the temperature of liquids used in your recipes, ensuring they are not too hot or too cold for the yeast.

Additional Tools and Accessories

> Mixing Bowls: For preparing your sourdough starter and pre-mixing dry ingredients.

> Silicone Spatula: To help mix and scrape down the sides of the bread machine pan.

> Bread Pan Liners or Parchment Paper: Useful for preventing sticking and for easy removal of bread from the pan.

➢ Wire Rack: For cooling your bread post-baking to avoid sogginess.

This chapter layed the foundation for your gluten-free sourdough baking. By understanding and gathering these essential ingredients and tools, you're setting yourself up for success. Remember, the quality of your ingredients and the precision of your measurements play a significant role in the outcome of your bread. With these essentials, you're ready to dive into the world of gluten-free sourdough bread making, creating loaves that are not only delicious but also cater to your dietary needs.

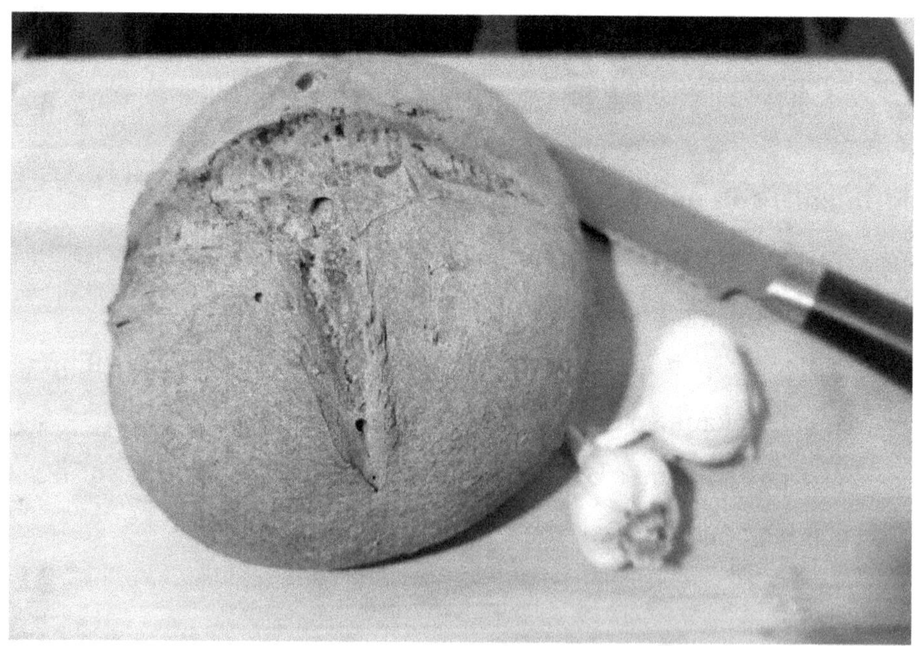

CHAPTER 3

Fundamentals of Sourdough Starter

The soul of every sourdough bread, whether classic or gluten-free, lies in its starter. This chapter will guide you through creating and maintaining a gluten-free sourdough starter, ensuring that even beginners can confidently embark on this essential step in sourdough baking.

Creating Your Gluten-Free Sourdough Starter

1. Choosing Your Flour: Begin with a gluten-free flour blend or a single gluten-free flour like brown rice flour. These flours are not just gluten-free; they are also excellent for fermentation.

2. Mixing with Water: Combine equal parts (by weight) of your gluten-free flour and water. Use non-chlorinated water to ensure that the natural yeasts aren't inhibited.

3. Consistency: Aim for a consistency like thick pancake batter. This allows the yeast to move and feed easily.

4. Feeding Routine: Feed your starter daily with equal parts of gluten-free flour and water. In a week, your starter should show signs of life: bubbling and a slightly sour smell.

5. Storing Your Starter: Once active, store your starter in the refrigerator and feed it once a week.

Maintaining Your Sourdough Starter

- Regular Feeding: Even if stored in the fridge, your starter needs regular feeding. A well-fed starter is the key to great sourdough bread.

- Observing Changes: Your starter will grow and bubble a few hours after feeding, indicating good health.

- Discarding: When feeding your starter, discard a portion before adding fresh flour and water. This keeps the yeast vigorous and not overwhelmed.

- Reviving a Neglected Starter: If your starter seems sluggish, increase feedings to twice a day at room temperature until it becomes active again.

Troubleshooting Common Issues

- No Bubbles: If your starter isn't bubbling after a few days, try moving it to a warmer spot and ensure you're using non-chlorinated water.

- Mold Growth: If you see any signs of mold, it's best to discard the starter and begin anew. Mold indicates contamination.

- Too Sour or Not Sour Enough: Adjust the frequency of feedings. Less frequent feedings increase sourness, while more frequent feedings decrease it.

- Liquid Layer (Hooch): A layer of liquid on top of your starter is normal, especially in the fridge. You can stir it back in or pour it off before feeding.

CHAPTER 4

Classic Gluten-Free Sourdough Recipes

Basic Gluten-Free Sourdough Loaf

Ingredients:

- 1 cup gluten-free sourdough starter
- 3 cups gluten-free flour blend
- 1 ¼ cups warm water
- 2 tsp sugar
- 2 tsp salt
- 2 tbsp olive oil
- 1 tsp xanthan gum (if not in your flour blend)

Instructions:

1. Combine all ingredients in the bread machine pan.
2. Select the gluten-free setting on your bread machine.
3. Start the bread machine and let it run through the cycle.
4. Once done, remove the loaf and let it cool on a wire rack.

- Prep Time: 10 minutes + baking time in the bread machine.
- Servings: 1 loaf (approximately 12 slices)

Nutritional Information: (Per slice) Calories: 150, Protein: 3g, Fat: 2.5g, Carbohydrates: 28g

Multigrain Sourdough

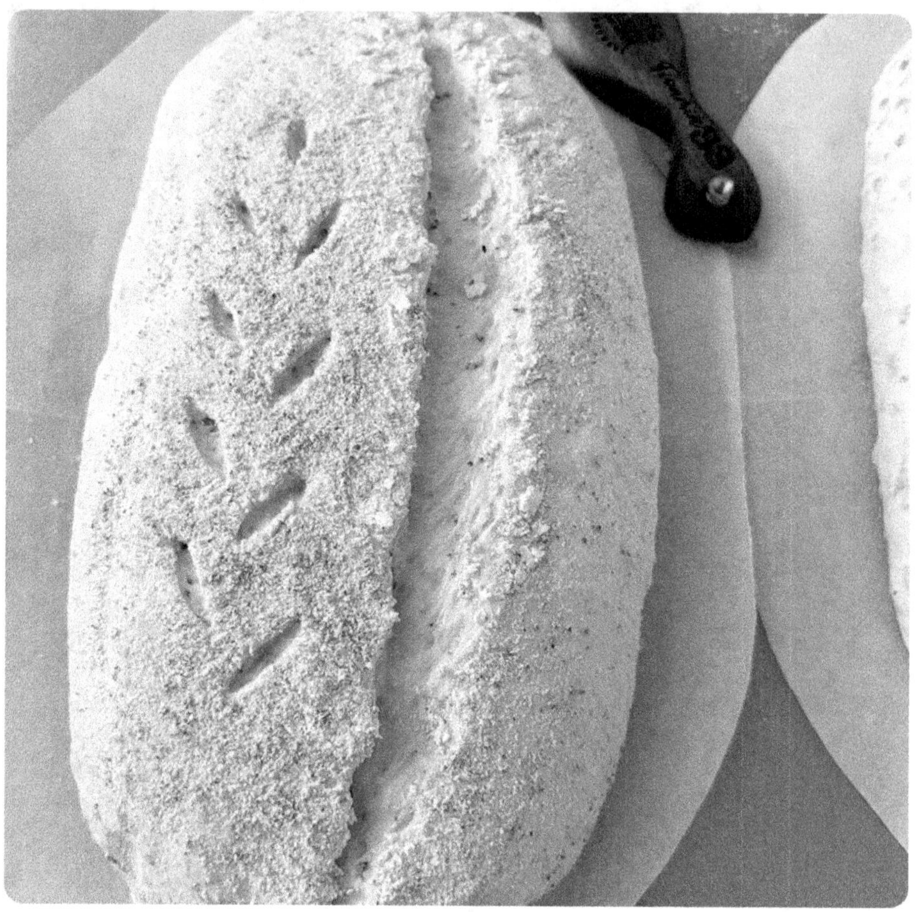

Ingredients:

- 1 cup gluten-free sourdough starter
- 2 cups gluten-free multigrain flour blend
- 1 cup brown rice flour
- 1 ½ cups warm water
- 2 tbsp honey

- 2 tsp salt
- 2 tbsp vegetable oil
- 1 tsp xanthan gum (if not in your flour blend)

Instructions:

1. Add all ingredients to the bread machine pan in the order recommended by the manufacturer.
2. Select the gluten-free setting.
3. Start the machine and let it complete the cycle.
4. Remove the loaf and let it cool before slicing.

- o Prep Time: 10 minutes + baking time.
- o Servings: 1 loaf

Nutritional Information: (Per slice) Calories: 160, Protein: 4g, Fat: 3g, Carbohydrates: 30g

Rustic Sourdough Baguette

Ingredients:

- 1 cup gluten-free sourdough starter
- 2 ½ cups gluten-free flour blend
- 1 ¼ cups warm water
- 1 tsp salt
- 1 tbsp sugar
- 2 tbsp olive oil
- 1 tsp xanthan gum (if not in your flour blend)

Instructions:

1. Combine ingredients in the bread machine pan.

2. Use the dough setting on your bread machine.

3. Once the dough cycle is complete, shape the dough into a baguette form.

4. Bake in a preheated oven at 375°F (190°C) for 25-30 minutes.

5. Let it cool on a wire rack.

   o Prep Time: 15 minutes + baking and cooling time.

   o Servings: 1 baguette

Nutritional Information: (Per slice) Calories: 140, Protein: 3g, Fat: 2g, Carbohydrates: 27g

Gluten-Free Sourdough Pancakes

Ingredients:

- 2 cups gluten-free sourdough starter
- 1 egg
- 2 tbsp melted butter or oil
- 1 tsp baking soda
- ½ tsp salt
- 1 tbsp sugar or honey
- ½ cup milk or milk alternative

Instructions:

1. In a bowl, combine all ingredients and mix until smooth.

2. Heat a griddle or pan over medium heat.

3. Pour ¼ cup of batter for each pancake.

4. Cook until bubbles form, then flip and cook the other side.

5. Serve hot.

- o   Prep Time: 10 minutes

- o   Servings: 4 servings (2 pancakes each)

Nutritional Information: (Per serving) Calories: 210, Protein: 6g, Fat: 8g, Carbohydrates: 30g

Gluten-Free Sourdough Chocolate Bread

Ingredients:

- 1 cup gluten-free sourdough starter

- 2 ½ cups gluten-free flour blend

- 1 cup warm water

- ½ cup cocoa powder

- ¾ cup sugar

- 2 tsp vanilla extract

- ½ cup melted butter

- 1 tsp xanthan gum (if not in your flour blend)

Instructions:

1. Add all ingredients to the bread machine pan.

2. Select the gluten-free setting.

3. Start the machine and let it complete the cycle.

4. Remove the bread and let it cool on a wire rack.

o   Prep Time: 10 minutes + baking time.

o   Servings: 1 loaf

Nutritional Information: (Per slice) Calories: 180, Protein: 3g, Fat: 7g, Carbohydrates: 29g

Gluten-Free Sourdough Fruit Loaf

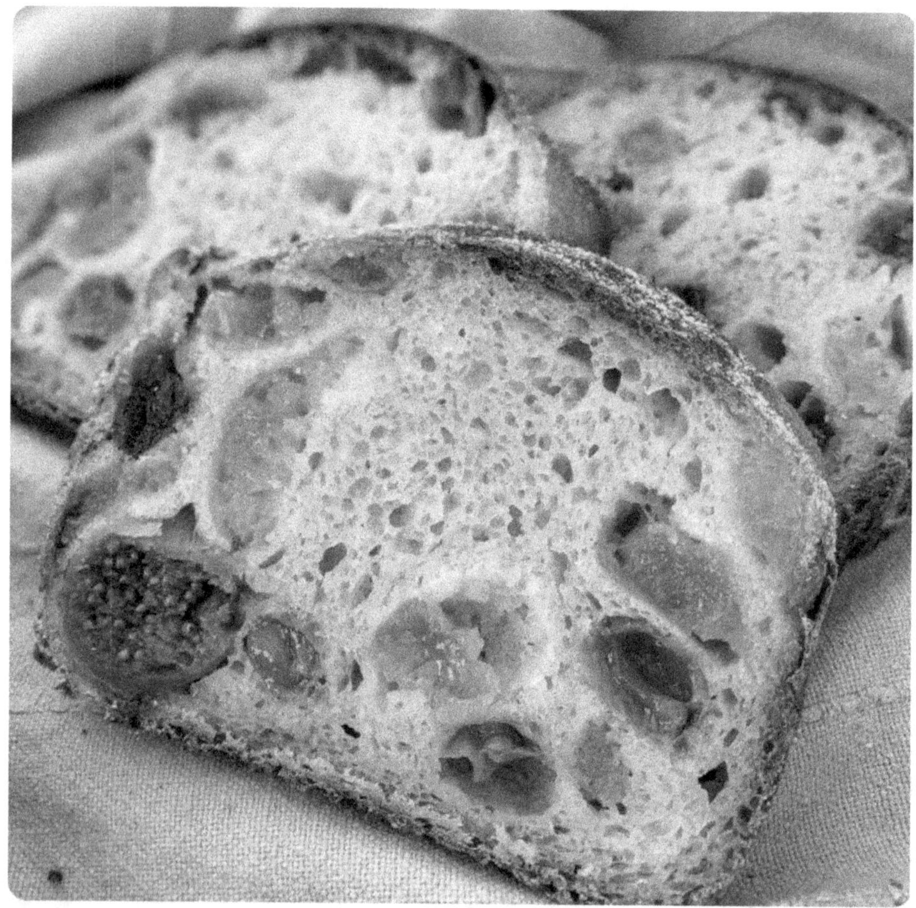

Ingredients:

- 1 cup gluten-free sourdough starter
- 3 cups gluten-free flour blend
- 1 ¼ cups warm water
- ¼ cup honey
- ½ cup mixed dried fruits (raisins, apricots, etc.)
- 2 tsp cinnamon
- 1 tsp xanthan gum (if not in your flour blend)

Instructions:

1. Combine all ingredients in the bread machine pan.
2. Use the gluten-free setting on your bread machine.
3. Once the cycle is complete, remove the loaf and cool.
   - Prep Time: 10 minutes + baking time.
   - Servings: 1 loaf

Nutritional Information: (Per slice) Calories: 160, Protein: 3g, Fat: 1g, Carbohydrates: 35g

Gluten-Free Sourdough Dinner Rolls

Ingredients:

- 1 cup gluten-free sourdough starter
- 2 ½ cups gluten-free flour blend
- 1 cup warm milk (dairy or plant-based)
- 2 tbsp sugar
- 2 tbsp melted butter
- 1 tsp salt

- 1 tsp xanthan gum (if not in your flour blend)

Instructions:

1. Mix ingredients in the bread machine using the dough setting.
2. Once the dough is ready, shape into rolls.
3. Place on a baking tray and let rest for 30 minutes.
4. Bake at 350°F (175°C) for 20 minutes or until golden.
   - Prep Time: 20 minutes + baking time.
   - Servings: 12 rolls

Nutritional Information: (Per roll) Calories: 150, Protein: 3g, Fat: 3g, Carbohydrates: 28g

Gluten-Free Sourdough Garlic & Herb Bread

Ingredients:

- 1 cup gluten-free sourdough starter
- 3 cups gluten-free flour blend
- 1 ¼ cups warm water
- 1/4 cup olive oil
- 3 cloves garlic, minced
- 2 tsp dried Italian herbs
- 1 tsp xanthan gum (if not in your flour blend)

Instructions:

1. Combine all ingredients in the bread machine pan.
2. Select the gluten-free setting.

3. After baking, let the bread cool before slicing.

- o Prep Time: 10 minutes + baking time.
- o Servings: 1 loaf

Nutritional Information: (Per slice) Calories: 160, Protein: 3g, Fat: 5g, Carbohydrates: 27g

Gluten-Free Sourdough Rye-Style Bread

Ingredients:

- 1 cup gluten-free sourdough starter
- 2 cups gluten-free flour blend
- 1 cup buckwheat flour
- 1 ½ cups warm water
- 2 tbsp molasses
- 1 tsp caraway seeds
- 1 tsp xanthan gum (if not in your flour blend)

Instructions:

1. Add all ingredients to the bread machine pan.
2. Use the gluten-free setting.
3. Once baked, allow to cool before slicing.

- o Prep Time: 10 minutes + baking time.
- o Servings: 1 loaf

Nutritional Information: (Per slice) Calories: 160, Protein: 4g, Fat: 1g, Carbohydrates: 34g

Gluten-Free Sourdough Olive Bread

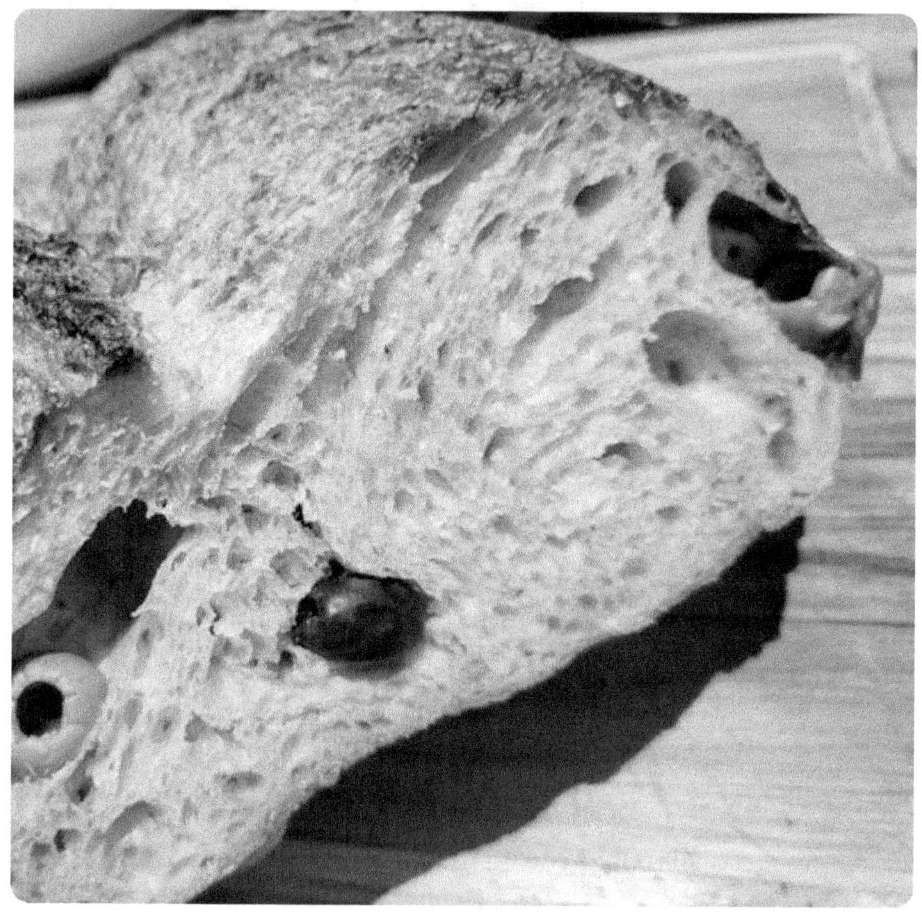

Ingredients:

- 1 cup gluten-free sourdough starter
- 3 cups gluten-free flour blend
- 1 ¼ cups warm water
- 1/3 cup chopped olives (green or black)
- 2 tbsp olive oil

- 1 tsp salt
- 1 tsp xanthan gum (if not in your flour blend)

Instructions:

1. Mix all ingredients in the bread machine pan.
2. Select the gluten-free setting.
3. After the cycle, cool the bread on a wire rack.

- Prep Time: 10 minutes + baking time.
- Servings: 1 loaf

Nutritional Information: (Per slice) Calories: 170, Protein: 3g, Fat: 4g, Carbohydrates: 30g

Gluten-Free Sourdough Walnut Bread

Ingredients:

- 1 cup gluten-free sourdough starter
- 2 ½ cups gluten-free flour blend
- 1 cup warm water
- ½ cup chopped walnuts
- 3 tbsp maple syrup
- 1 tsp salt
- 1 tsp xanthan gum (if not in your flour blend)

Instructions:

1. Add all ingredients to your bread machine pan.
2. Use the gluten-free setting.
3. Once baked, let the bread cool before slicing.

- o   Prep Time: 10 minutes + baking time.
- o   Servings: 1 loaf

Nutritional Information: (Per slice) Calories: 180, Protein: 4g, Fat: 6g, Carbohydrates: 30g

Gluten-Free Sourdough Banana Bread

Ingredients:

- 1 cup gluten-free sourdough starter
- 2 cups gluten-free flour blend
- 3 ripe bananas, mashed
- ¾ cup sugar
- ½ cup vegetable oil
- 2 eggs
- 1 tsp vanilla extract
- 1 tsp baking soda
- 1 tsp xanthan gum (if not in your flour blend)

Instructions:

1. Combine all ingredients in the bread machine pan.
2. Select the gluten-free setting.
3. After baking, let the bread cool before serving.

- o   Prep Time: 15 minutes + baking time.
- o   Servings: 1 loaf

Nutritional Information: (Per slice) Calories: 200, Protein: 3g, Fat: 8g, Carbohydrates: 32g

Gluten-Free Sourdough Hotcakes

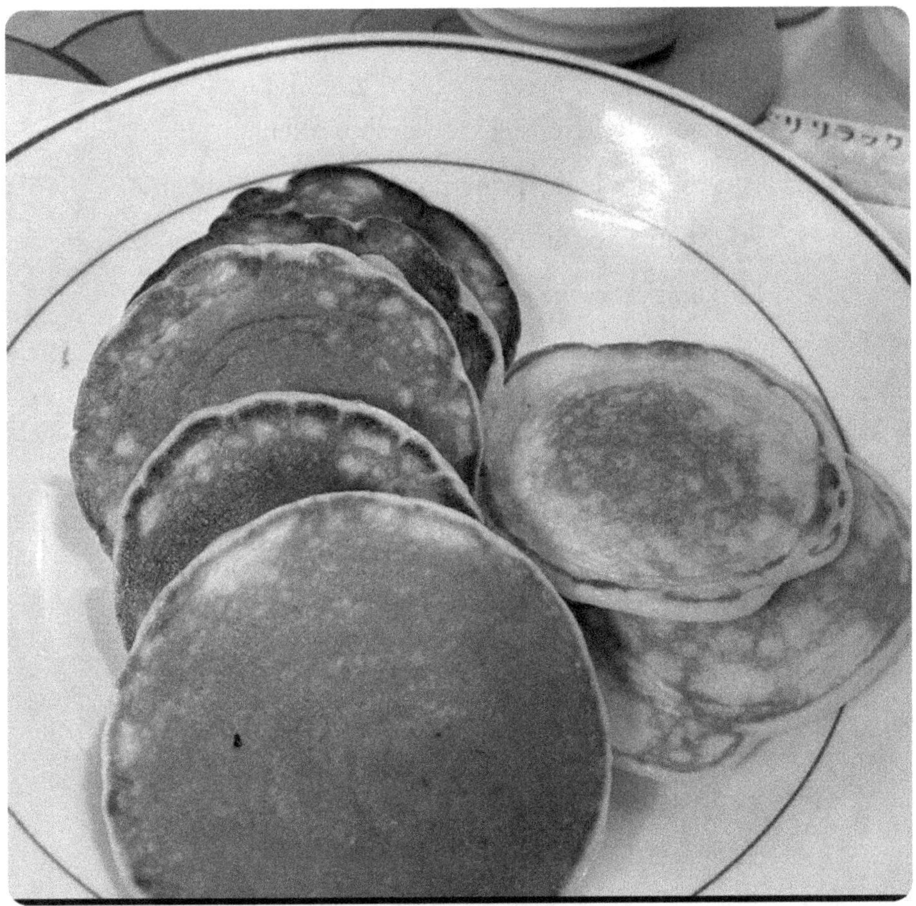

Ingredients:

- 2 cups gluten-free sourdough discard
- 1 egg
- 2 tbsp melted butter or oil
- 1 tsp baking soda
- ½ tsp salt

- 1 tbsp sugar or honey

- ½ cup milk or alternative

Instructions:

1. In a bowl, whisk together all ingredients.

2. Heat a griddle or frying pan over medium heat.

3. Pour batter to form hotcakes and cook until bubbles appear.

4. Flip and cook the other side.

5. Serve warm with your favorite toppings.

- o Prep Time: 10 minutes

- o Servings: 4 (2 hotcakes each)

Nutritional Information: (Per serving) Calories: 210, Protein: 5g, Fat: 9g, Carbohydrates: 28g

Gluten-Free Sourdough Griddle Cakes

Ingredients:

- 2 cups gluten-free sourdough discard

- 2 eggs

- 3 tbsp melted butter or oil

- 1 tsp vanilla extract

- ½ tsp cinnamon

- 1 tsp baking powder

- 2 tbsp maple syrup

- Butter or oil for the griddle

Instructions:

1. Combine all ingredients in a bowl and mix until smooth.

2. Preheat a griddle or skillet and lightly grease.

3. Pour the batter to form griddle cakes. Cook until golden.

4. Flip and cook the other side.

5. Serve hot with your choice of toppings.

- Prep Time: 10 minutes
- Servings: 4-6

Nutritional Information: (Per serving) Calories: 220, Protein: 6g, Fat: 10g, Carbohydrates: 28g

Gluten-Free Sourdough Seed & Nut Loaf

Ingredients:

1. 1 cup gluten-free sourdough starter

2. 2 ½ cups gluten-free flour blend

3. 1 cup warm water

4. ¼ cup mixed seeds (sunflower, pumpkin, etc.)

5. ¼ cup chopped nuts (almonds, walnuts, etc.)

6. 2 tbsp honey

7. 1 tsp xanthan gum (if not in your flour blend)

Instructions:

1. Mix all ingredients in the bread machine pan.

2. Choose the gluten-free setting.

3. After the baking cycle, cool the loaf before slicing.

o   Prep Time: 10 minutes + baking time.

o   Servings: 1 loaf

Nutritional Information: (Per slice) Calories: 170, Protein:

Each recipe in this chapter has been thoughtfully crafted, keeping in mind the nuances of gluten-free baking. Unlike traditional wheat-based sourdough, gluten-free dough typically does not have a second rise, so the recipes are designed to work beautifully without this step. Enjoy the process of creating these delicious, gluten-free sourdough treats that are perfect for any occasion.

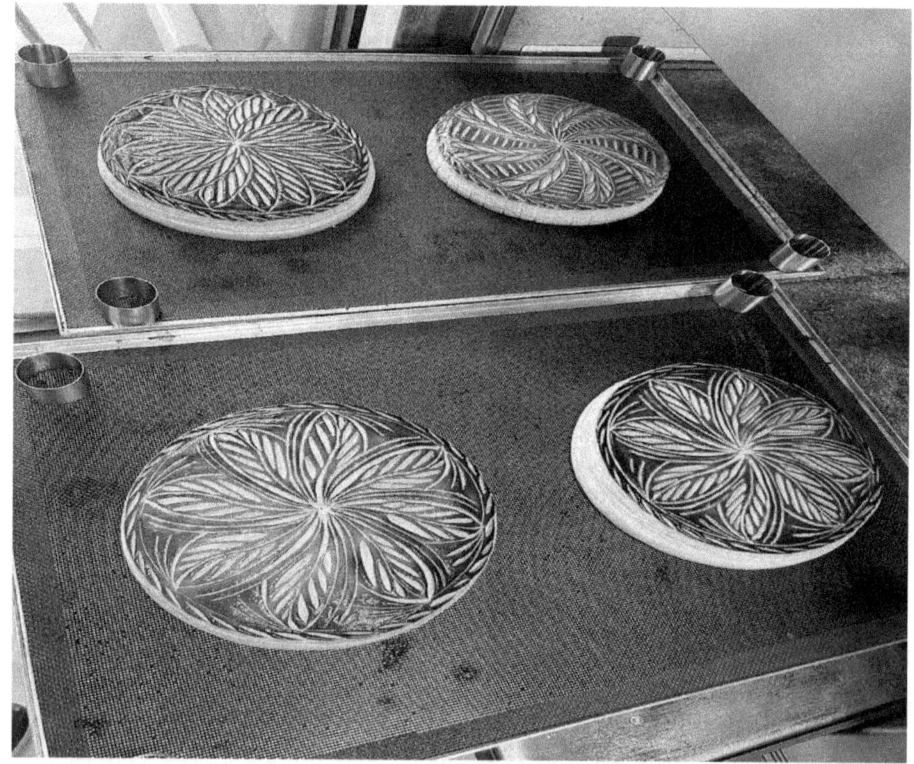

CHAPTER 5

Sweet and Savory Variations

Gluten-Free Sourdough Cinnamon Raisin Bread

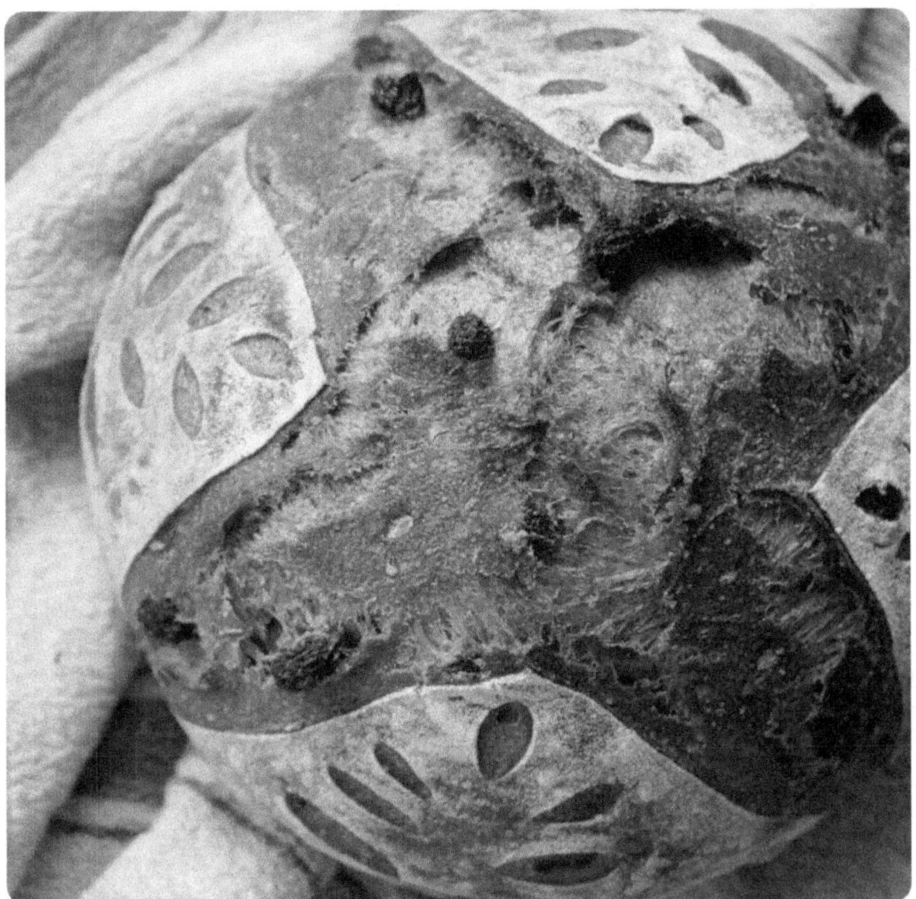

Ingredients:

- 1 cup sourdough starter (gluten-free)

- 2 cups gluten-free flour blend
- 1 tsp salt
- 1/4 cup sugar
- 2 tsp cinnamon
- 1/2 cup raisins
- 1 cup water
- 2 tbsp vegetable oil

Instructions:

1. Combine all dry ingredients except raisins in the bread machine pan.
2. Add water, vegetable oil, and sourdough starter.
3. Set your bread machine to the gluten-free setting.
4. Add raisins when the mix-in tone sounds.
5. Let the bread machine complete the cycle.

- Prep Time: 10 minutes
- Cook Time: Depends on bread machine
- Servings: 1 loaf

Nutritional Information: (per slice) Calories: 180, Fat: 3g, Carbs: 35g, Protein: 3g

Olive and Rosemary Sourdough

Ingredients:

- 1 cup sourdough starter (gluten-free)
- 2 cups gluten-free flour blend

- 1 tsp salt
- 1/4 cup chopped black olives
- 2 tbsp fresh rosemary, chopped
- 1 cup water
- 2 tbsp olive oil

Instructions:

1. Add water, olive oil, and sourdough starter to the bread machine pan.
2. Mix in the gluten-free flour blend, salt, olives, and rosemary.
3. Choose the gluten-free setting on your bread machine.
4. Start the cycle and let the bread machine do the work.

- o Prep Time: 10 minutes
- o Cook Time: Depends on bread machine
- o Servings: 1 loaf

Nutritional Information: (per slice) Calories: 190, Fat: 4g, Carbs: 34g, Protein: 4g

Sun-Dried Tomato and Basil Sourdough

Ingredients:

- 1 cup sourdough starter (gluten-free)
- 2 cups gluten-free flour blend
- 1 tsp salt
- 1/4 cup sun-dried tomatoes, chopped

- 2 tbsp fresh basil, chopped
- 1 cup water
- 2 tbsp olive oil

Instructions:

1. Place water, olive oil, and sourdough starter into the bread machine pan.
2. Add the gluten-free flour, salt, sun-dried tomatoes, and basil.
3. Set the bread machine to the gluten-free setting.
4. Start the cycle and wait for your delicious bread.

- o Prep Time: 10 minutes
- o Cook Time: Depends on bread machine
- o Servings: 1 loaf

Nutritional Information: (per slice) Calories: 200, Fat: 4.5g, Carbs: 36g, Protein: 4g

Gluten-Free Sourdough Garlic Herb Bread

Ingredients:

- 1 cup gluten-free sourdough starter
- 2 cups gluten-free flour blend
- 1 tsp salt
- 1 tbsp sugar
- 1 tsp garlic powder

- 2 tbsp mixed dried herbs (such as thyme, oregano, and rosemary)
- 1 cup water
- 2 tbsp olive oil

Instructions:

1. Place water, olive oil, and sourdough starter into the bread machine pan.
2. Add the gluten-free flour, salt, sugar, garlic powder, and mixed herbs.
3. Set the bread machine to the gluten-free setting.
4. Start the cycle; once done, let the bread cool on a wire rack.

   o Prep Time: 10 minutes
   o Cook Time: Depends on bread machine
   o Servings: 1 loaf

Nutritional Information: (per slice) Calories: 180, Fat: 3.5g, Carbs: 33g, Protein: 3g

Gluten-Free Sourdough Apple Cinnamon Bread

Ingredients:

- 1 cup gluten-free sourdough starter
- 2 cups gluten-free flour blend
- 1 tsp salt
- 1/4 cup sugar
- 2 tsp cinnamon

- 1 cup finely chopped apple
- 1 cup water
- 2 tbsp vegetable oil

Instructions:

1. Combine all dry ingredients except apple in the bread machine pan.
2. Add water, vegetable oil, and sourdough starter.
3. Set your bread machine to the gluten-free setting.
4. Add chopped apple when the mix-in tone sounds.
5. Let the bread machine complete the cycle.

Prep Time: 15 minutes

Cook Time: Depends on bread machine

Servings: 1 loaf

Nutritional Information: (per slice) Calories: 190, Fat: 3g, Carbs: 37g, Protein: 3g

Gluten-Free Sourdough Cheese and Onion Bread

Ingredients:

- 1 cup gluten-free sourdough starter
- 2 cups gluten-free flour blend
- 1 tsp salt
- 1/2 cup grated cheese (cheddar or your preference)
- 1/4 cup finely chopped onion
- 1 cup water

- 2 tbsp olive oil

Instructions:

1. Place water, olive oil, and sourdough starter into the bread machine pan.
2. Add the gluten-free flour, salt, cheese, and onion.
3. Set the bread machine to the gluten-free setting.
4. Start the cycle; once done, let the bread cool before slicing.

Prep Time: 15 minutes

Cook Time: Depends on bread machine

Servings: 1 loaf

Nutritional Information: (per slice) Calories: 210, Fat: 6g, Carbs: 34g, Protein: 5g

Gluten-Free Sourdough Chocolate Chip Bread

Ingredients:

- 1 cup gluten-free sourdough starter
- 2 cups gluten-free flour blend
- 1 tsp salt
- 1/4 cup sugar
- 1/2 cup chocolate chips
- 1 cup water
- 2 tbsp vegetable oil

Instructions:

1. Combine dry ingredients, except chocolate chips, in the bread machine pan.
2. Add water, vegetable oil, and sourdough starter.
3. Set your bread machine to the gluten-free setting.
4. Add chocolate chips when the mix-in tone sounds.
5. Complete the cycle and cool the bread on a wire rack.

- o Prep Time: 10 minutes
- o Cook Time: Depends on bread machine
- o Servings: 1 loaf

Nutritional Information: (per slice) Calories: 200, Fat: 5g, Carbs: 36g, Protein: 3g

Gluten-Free Sourdough Walnut and Cranberry Bread

Ingredients:

- 1 cup gluten-free sourdough starter
- 2 cups gluten-free flour blend
- 1 tsp salt
- 1/4 cup sugar
- 1/2 cup dried cranberries
- 1/2 cup chopped walnuts
- 1 cup water
- 2 tbsp vegetable oil

Instructions:

1. Add dry ingredients, except cranberries and walnuts, to the bread machine pan.

2. Incorporate water, vegetable oil, and sourdough starter.

3. Select the gluten-free setting on your bread machine.

4. Add cranberries and walnuts when the mix-in tone sounds.

5. Complete the baking cycle and cool the bread on a rack.

o   Prep Time: 10 minutes

o   Cook Time: Depends on bread machine

o   Servings: 1 loaf

Nutritional Information: (per slice) Calories: 210, Fat: 6g, Carbs: 35g, Protein: 4g

Gluten-Free Sourdough Olive and Feta Bread

Ingredients:

- 1 cup gluten-free sourdough starter
- 2 cups gluten-free flour blend
- 1 tsp salt
- 1/2 cup chopped kalamata olives
- 1/2 cup crumbled feta cheese
- 1 cup water
- 2 tbsp olive oil

Instructions:

1. Combine water, olive oil, and sourdough starter in the bread machine pan.

2. Add flour, salt, olives, and feta cheese.

3. Set the machine to the gluten-free setting.

4. Start the cycle and let the machine complete the baking process.

- o Prep Time: 15 minutes
- o Cook Time: Depends on bread machine
- o Servings: 1 loaf

Nutritional Information: (per slice) Calories: 220, Fat: 7g, Carbs: 33g, Protein: 5g

Gluten-Free Sourdough Pumpkin Spice Bread

Ingredients:

- 1 cup gluten-free sourdough starter
- 2 cups gluten-free flour blend
- 1 tsp salt
- 1/4 cup sugar
- 2 tsp pumpkin spice mix
- 1/2 cup pumpkin puree
- 1 cup water
- 2 tbsp vegetable oil

Instructions:

1. Add water, pumpkin puree, vegetable oil, and sourdough starter to the bread machine pan.

2. Mix in the flour, salt, sugar, and pumpkin spice.

3. Choose the gluten-free setting on your bread machine.

4. Start the cycle; once complete, allow the bread to cool.

o   Prep Time: 15 minutes

o   Cook Time: Depends on bread machine

o   Servings: 1 loaf

Nutritional Information: (per slice) Calories: 200, Fat: 4g, Carbs: 37g, Protein: 3g

Gluten-Free Sourdough Chocolate Hazelnut Bread

Ingredients:

- 1 cup gluten-free sourdough starter
- 2 cups gluten-free flour blend
- 1 tsp salt
- 1/4 cup sugar
- 1/2 cup chopped hazelnuts
- 1/2 cup chocolate chips
- 1 cup water
- 2 tbsp vegetable oil

Instructions:

1. Mix dry ingredients, except hazelnuts and chocolate chips, in the bread machine pan.

2. Add water, vegetable oil, and sourdough starter.

3. Set your bread machine to the gluten-free setting.

4. Add hazelnuts and chocolate chips when the mix-in tone sounds.

5. Let the machine complete the baking cycle.

   o Prep Time: 10 minutes

   o Cook Time: Depends on bread machine

   o Servings: 1 loaf

Nutritional Information: (per slice) Calories: 220, Fat: 7g, Carbs: 35g, Protein: 4g

Gluten-Free Sourdough Banana Nut Bread

Ingredients:

- 1 cup gluten-free sourdough starter
- 2 cups gluten-free flour blend
- 1 tsp salt
- 1/4 cup sugar
- 1/2 cup mashed ripe banana
- 1/2 cup chopped walnuts
- 1 cup water
- 2 tbsp vegetable oil

Instructions:

1. In the bread machine pan, combine water, vegetable oil, sourdough starter, and mashed banana.

2. Add the gluten-free flour, salt, and sugar.

3. Set the machine to the gluten-free setting.

4. Add walnuts when the mix-in tone sounds.

5. Once the cycle is complete, remove and let the bread cool.

   o Prep Time: 15 minutes

   o Cook Time: Depends on bread machine

   o Servings: 1 loaf

Nutritional Information: (per slice) Calories: 210, Fat: 6g, Carbs: 36g, Protein: 4g

Gluten-Free Sourdough Parmesan and Black Pepper Bread

Ingredients:

- 1 cup gluten-free sourdough starter
- 2 cups gluten-free flour blend
- 1 tsp salt
- 1/2 cup grated Parmesan cheese
- 1 tsp ground black pepper
- 1 cup water
- 2 tbsp olive oil

Instructions:

1. Place water, olive oil, and sourdough starter in the bread machine pan.

2. Add the gluten-free flour, salt, Parmesan cheese, and black pepper.

3. Select the gluten-free setting on your bread machine.

4. Start the cycle and let the machine complete the baking process.

- o Prep Time: 10 minutes
- o Cook Time: Depends on bread machine
- o Servings: 1 loaf

Nutritional Information: (per slice) Calories: 220, Fat: 7g, Carbs: 33g, Protein: 6g

Gluten-Free Sourdough Blueberry Lemon Bread

Ingredients:

- 1 cup gluten-free sourdough starter
- 2 cups gluten-free flour blend
- 1 tsp salt
- 1/4 cup sugar
- 1/2 cup fresh blueberries
- Zest of 1 lemon
- 1 cup water
- 2 tbsp vegetable oil

Instructions:

1. Combine water, vegetable oil, sourdough starter, and lemon zest in the bread machine pan.
2. Add in the gluten-free flour, salt, and sugar.
3. Set your bread machine to the gluten-free setting.
4. Gently add blueberries when the mix-in tone sounds.

5. Complete the baking cycle and let the bread cool before slicing.

- o Prep Time: 10 minutes
- o Cook Time: Depends on bread machine
- o Servings: 1 loaf

Nutritional Information: (per slice) Calories: 200, Fat: 4g, Carbs: 37g, Protein: 3g

Gluten-Free Sourdough Jalapeño Cheddar Bread

Ingredients:

- 1 cup gluten-free sourdough starter
- 2 cups gluten-free flour blend
- 1 tsp salt
- 1/2 cup shredded cheddar cheese
- 1/4 cup diced jalapeños (adjust to taste)
- 1 cup water
- 2 tbsp olive oil

Instructions:

1. Add water, olive oil, and sourdough starter to the bread machine pan.
2. Mix in the flour, salt, cheddar cheese, and jalapeños.
3. Choose the gluten-free setting on your bread machine.
4. Start the cycle; once done, let the bread cool before serving.

- o Prep Time: 10 minutes

- o Cook Time: Depends on bread machine
- o Servings: 1 loaf

Nutritional Information: (per slice) Calories: 215, Fat: 7g, Carbs: 32g, Protein: 5g

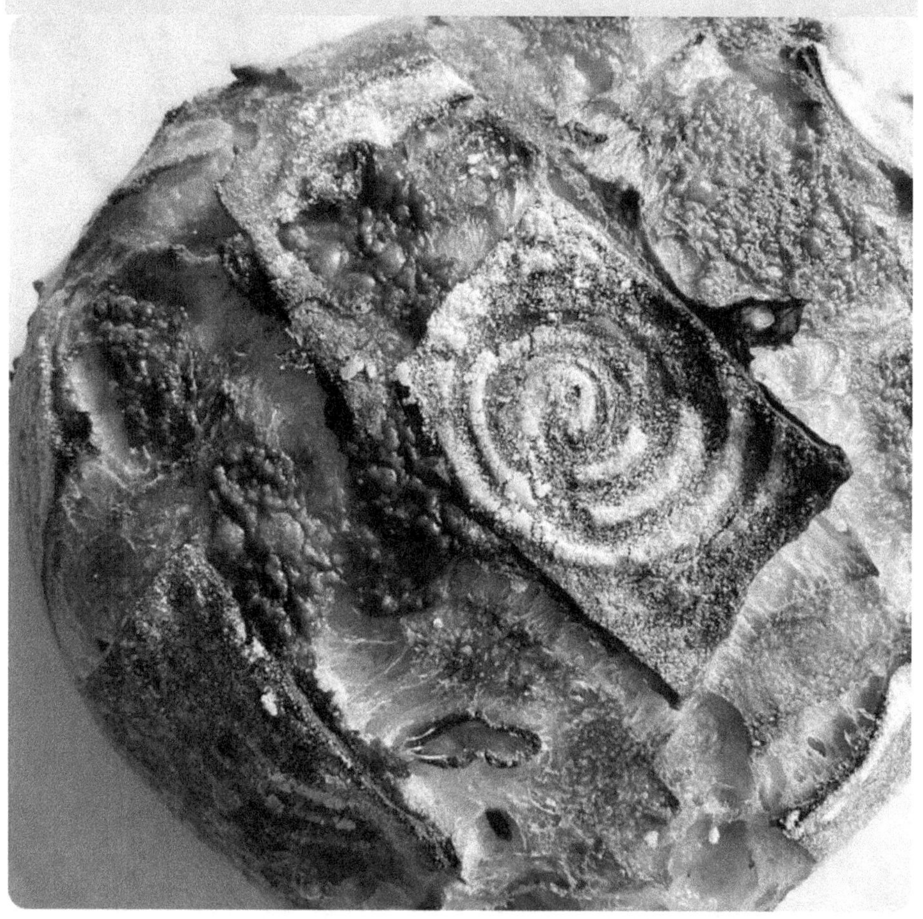

Jalapeño Cheddar Bread

Specialty Sourdough Delights

Gluten-Free Sourdough Focaccia

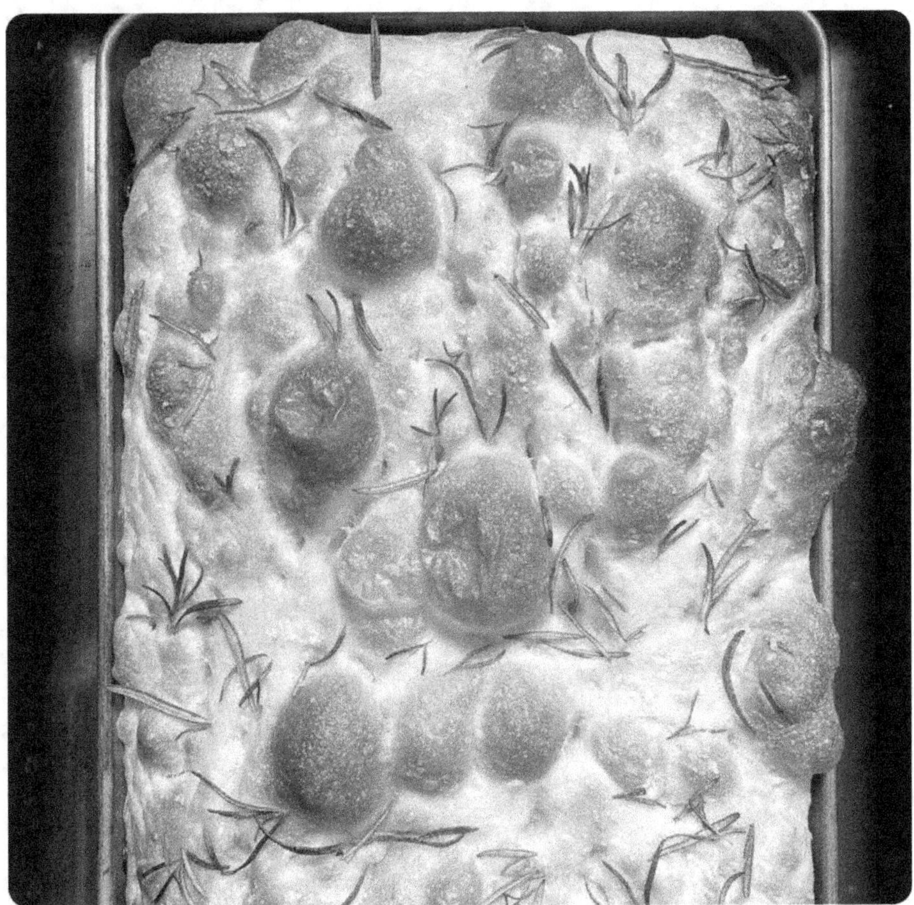

Ingredients:

- 1 cup gluten-free sourdough starter

- 3 cups gluten-free flour blend
- 1 tsp salt
- 1 tsp sugar
- 1 1/2 cups water
- 1/4 cup olive oil, plus more for drizzling
- Fresh rosemary and sea salt for topping

Instructions:

1. Combine the starter, flour, salt, sugar, water, and 1/4 cup olive oil in the bread machine pan.
2. Use the dough setting on your bread machine.
3. Once the dough is ready, spread it onto a greased baking tray.
4. Drizzle with olive oil, sprinkle with rosemary and sea salt.
5. Bake in a preheated oven at 400°F (200°C) for 20-25 minutes or until golden.

- o Prep Time: 20 minutes (excluding bread machine time)
- o Cook Time: 20-25 minutes
- o Servings: 8-10

Nutritional Information: (per serving) Calories: 230, Fat: 9g, Carbs: 34g, Protein: 3g

Sourdough Pizza Crust

Ingredients:

- 1 cup gluten-free sourdough starter

- 2 1/2 cups gluten-free flour blend
- 1 tsp salt
- 1 tsp sugar
- 1 cup water
- 2 tbsp olive oil

Instructions:

1. Place starter, flour, salt, sugar, water, and olive oil in the bread machine pan.
2. Select the dough setting.
3. After the cycle, roll out the dough on a floured surface.
4. Transfer to a pizza stone or baking sheet.
5. Add your favorite toppings and bake at 450°F (230°C) for 15-20 minutes.

   o Prep Time: 15 minutes (excluding bread machine time)
   o Cook Time: 15-20 minutes
   o Servings: 2-3

Nutritional Information: (per serving, without toppings) Calories: 220, Fat: 6g, Carbs: 38g, Protein: 3g

Gluten-Free Sourdough Pretzels

Ingredients:

- 1 cup gluten-free sourdough starter
- 2 3/4 cups gluten-free flour blend
- 1 tsp salt

- 1 tbsp sugar
- 1 cup warm water
- 2 tbsp olive oil
- Baking soda for boiling
- Coarse salt for topping

Instructions:

1. Combine starter, flour, salt, sugar, warm water, and olive oil in the bread machine pan.
2. Use the dough setting.
3. Once ready, divide the dough into 8 pieces and roll each into a long rope.
4. Twist into a pretzel shape.
5. Boil in water with a little baking soda, then bake at 425°F (220°C) for 12-15 minutes.
6. Sprinkle with coarse salt before serving.

- Prep Time: 25 minutes (excluding bread machine time)
- Cook Time: 12-15 minutes
- Servings: 8 pretzels

Nutritional Information: (per pretzel) Calories: 210, Fat: 5g, Carbs: 37g, Protein: 4g

Gluten-Free Sourdough Bagels

Ingredients:

- 1 cup gluten-free sourdough starter

- 3 cups gluten-free flour blend

- 1 1/2 tsp salt

- 1 tbsp sugar

- 1 1/4 cups warm water

- 1 tbsp olive oil

- Boiling water with 1 tbsp sugar for boiling bagels

- Sesame seeds or poppy seeds for topping

Instructions:

1. Combine the starter, flour, salt, sugar, warm water, and oil in the bread machine pan. Select the dough setting.

2. Once the cycle is complete, divide the dough and shape into bagels.

3. Boil each bagel for 30 seconds per side in the sugar water.

4. Place on a baking sheet, sprinkle with seeds, and bake at 425°F (220°C) for 20-25 minutes.

   - Prep Time: 20 minutes (excluding bread machine time)
   - Cook Time: 20-25 minutes
   - Servings: 6 bagels

Nutritional Information: (per bagel) Calories: 250, Fat: 4g, Carbs: 48g, Protein: 5g

Gluten-Free Sourdough English Muffins

Ingredients:

- 1 cup gluten-free sourdough starter

- 2 1/2 cups gluten-free flour blend
- 1 tsp salt
- 1 tbsp sugar
- 1 cup milk (or dairy-free alternative)
- 2 tbsp butter (or vegan substitute), melted
- Cornmeal for dusting

Instructions:

1. Mix starter, flour, salt, sugar, milk, and melted butter in the bread machine. Use the dough setting.
2. On a cornmeal-dusted surface, roll out the dough and cut into rounds.
3. Cook on a hot griddle or skillet until browned on both sides.
4. Split and toast before serving.

- Prep Time: 15 minutes (excluding bread machine time)
- Cook Time: 10 minutes
- Servings: 8-10 English muffins

Nutritional Information: (per muffin) Calories: 180, Fat: 3g, Carbs: 34g, Protein: 3g

Gluten-Free Sourdough Cinnamon Rolls

Ingredients:

For Dough:

- 1 cup gluten-free sourdough starter
- 2 1/2 cups gluten-free flour blend

- 1 tsp salt

- 1/4 cup sugar

- 1 cup milk (or dairy-free alternative)

- 2 tbsp butter (or vegan substitute), melted

For Filling:

- 1/2 cup brown sugar

- 2 tbsp cinnamon

- 1/4 cup butter (or vegan substitute), softened

- For Icing:

- 1 cup powdered sugar

- 2 tbsp milk (or dairy-free alternative)

Instructions:

1. Prepare dough in bread machine using the dough setting.

2. Roll out the dough, spread with butter, and sprinkle brown sugar and cinnamon.

3. Roll up the dough and cut into slices. Place in a baking dish.

4. Bake at 350°F (175°C) for 25-30 minutes.

5. Mix powdered sugar and milk for icing and drizzle over warm rolls.

- Prep Time: 20 minutes (excluding bread machine time)

- Cook Time: 25-30 minutes

- Servings: 12 cinnamon rolls

Nutritional Information: (per roll) Calories: 260, Fat: 6g, Carbs: 48g, Protein: 3g

Gluten-Free Sourdough Garlic Breadsticks

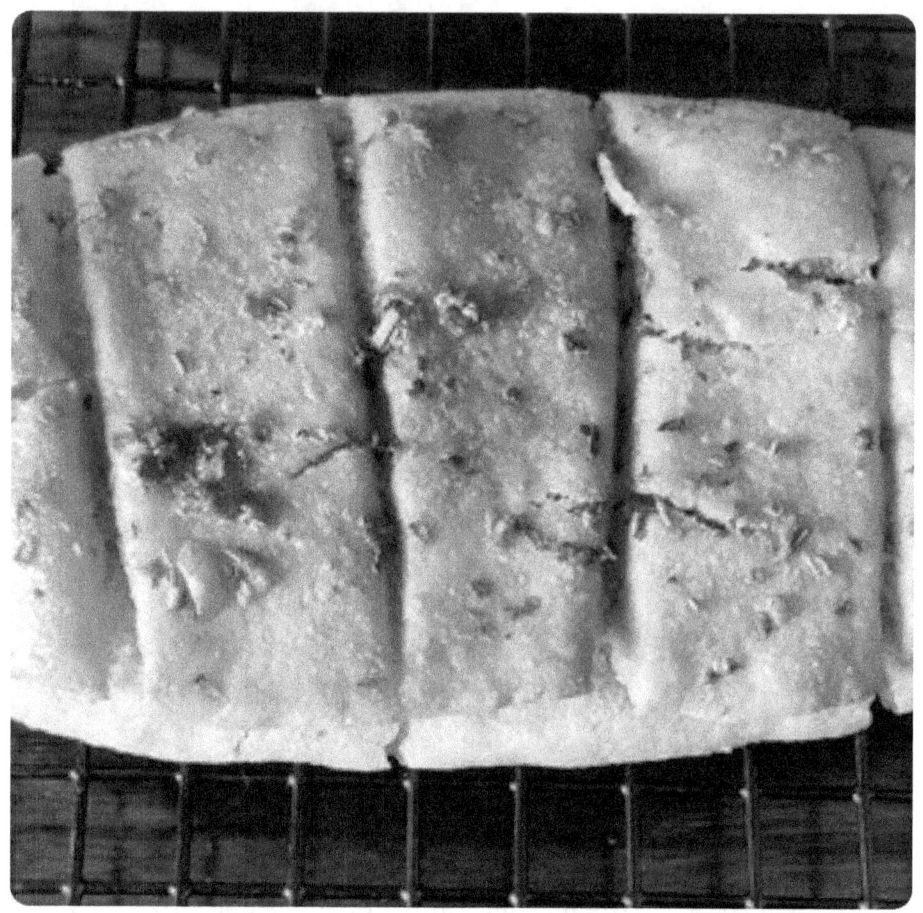

Ingredients:

- 1 cup gluten-free sourdough starter
- 2 3/4 cups gluten-free flour blend
- 1 tsp salt
- 1 tbsp sugar
- 1 cup warm water

- 2 tbsp olive oil

- 2 cloves garlic, minced

- 2 tbsp butter (or vegan substitute), melted

- 1 tbsp parsley, finely chopped

Instructions:

1. In the bread machine pan, combine starter, flour, salt, sugar, warm water, and oil using the dough setting.

2. Once the dough is ready, roll it out and cut into strips.

3. Place on a baking sheet, brush with garlic-infused melted butter, and sprinkle with parsley.

4. Bake at 400°F (200°C) for 15-20 minutes until golden.

- Prep Time: 20 minutes (excluding bread machine time)

- Cook Time: 15-20 minutes

- Servings: 12 breadsticks

Nutritional Information: (per breadstick) Calories: 180, Fat: 5g, Carbs: 30g, Protein: 3g

Gluten-Free Sourdough Herb and Cheese Rolls

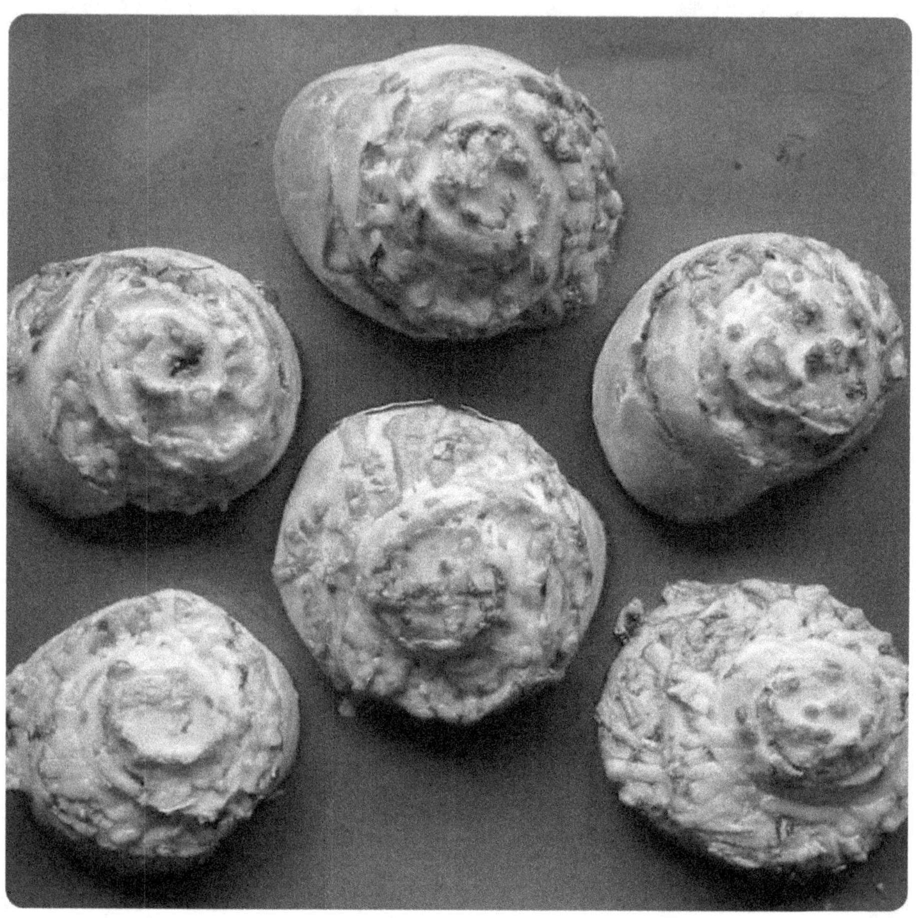

Ingredients:

- 1 cup gluten-free sourdough starter
- 3 cups gluten-free flour blend
- 1 tsp salt
- 1 tbsp sugar
- 1 cup warm water

- 2 tbsp olive oil
- 1/2 cup grated cheese (e.g., cheddar or mozzarella)
- 2 tbsp mixed herbs (e.g., thyme, rosemary, basil), chopped

Instructions:

1. Combine starter, flour, salt, sugar, warm water, and olive oil in the bread machine using the dough setting.
2. Once ready, divide the dough and form into rolls.
3. Press grated cheese and herbs onto the top of each roll.
4. Bake on a lined baking sheet at 375°F (190°C) for 20-25 minutes.

   o Prep Time: 20 minutes (excluding bread machine time)
   o Cook Time: 20-25 minutes
   o Servings: 12 rolls

Nutritional Information: (per roll) Calories: 210, Fat: 6g, Carbs: 34g, Protein: 5g

Gluten-Free Sourdough Pita Bread

Ingredients:

- 1 cup gluten-free sourdough starter
- 2 1/2 cups gluten-free flour blend
- 1 tsp salt
- 1 tbsp sugar
- 1 cup warm water
- 2 tbsp olive oil

Instructions:

1. In the bread machine pan, mix starter, flour, salt, sugar, warm water, and olive oil using the dough setting.
2. After the dough is ready, divide it and roll each piece into a circle.
3. Bake on a preheated pizza stone or a baking sheet at 425°F (220°C) for 7-10 minutes until puffed.

   o Prep Time: 15 minutes (excluding bread machine time)
   o Cook Time: 7-10 minutes
   o Servings: 6-8 pitas

Nutritional Information: (per pita) Calories: 200, Fat: 5g, Carbs: 35g, Protein: 3g

Gluten-Free Sourdough Rye-Style Bread

Ingredients:

- 1 cup gluten-free sourdough starter
- 2 cups gluten-free flour blend
- 1 cup buckwheat flour
- 1 tsp salt
- 1 tbsp molasses
- 1 tbsp caraway seeds
- 1 1/2 cups warm water
- 2 tbsp olive oil

Instructions:

1. Mix the starter, gluten-free flour blend, buckwheat flour, salt, molasses, caraway seeds, warm water, and olive oil in the bread machine using the dough setting.
2. After the cycle, shape the dough into a loaf and place in a greased loaf pan.
3. Bake at 375°F (190°C) for 35-40 minutes until the crust is dark and sounds hollow when tapped.

- Prep Time: 15 minutes (excluding bread machine time)
- Cook Time: 35-40 minutes
- Servings: 1 loaf

Nutritional Information: (per slice) Calories: 180, Fat: 4g, Carbs: 32g, Protein: 4g

Gluten-Free Sourdough Cranberry Walnut Loaf

Ingredients:

- 1 cup gluten-free sourdough starter
- 3 cups gluten-free flour blend
- 1 tsp salt
- 1/4 cup honey
- 1 cup dried cranberries
- 1/2 cup chopped walnuts
- 1 1/2 cups warm water
- 2 tbsp olive oil

Instructions:

1. Combine starter, flour, salt, honey, cranberries, walnuts, warm water, and oil in the bread machine on the dough setting.
2. Shape the dough into a loaf and place in a greased loaf pan.
3. Bake at 375°F (190°C) for 30-35 minutes until golden brown.

- o Prep Time: 20 minutes (excluding bread machine time)
- o Cook Time: 30-35 minutes
- o Servings: 1 loaf

Nutritional Information: (per slice) Calories: 210, Fat: 6g, Carbs: 36g, Protein: 4g

Gluten-Free Sourdough Zucchini Bread

Ingredients:

- 1 cup gluten-free sourdough starter
- 2 1/2 cups gluten-free flour blend
- 1 tsp salt
- 1/2 cup sugar
- 1 cup grated zucchini (excess water squeezed out)
- 1 tsp vanilla extract
- 1/2 cup vegetable oil
- 2 eggs, beaten

Instructions:

1. In a bowl, combine starter, flour, salt, sugar, zucchini, vanilla extract, oil, and eggs.

2. Transfer mixture into the bread machine pan and set it to the dough setting.

3. Once the cycle is complete, pour the batter into a greased loaf pan.

4. Bake at 350°F (175°C) for 50-60 minutes until a toothpick comes out clean.

   o Prep Time: 20 minutes (excluding bread machine time)

   o Cook Time: 50-60 minutes

   o Servings: 1 loaf

Nutritional Information: (per slice) Calories: 220, Fat: 10g, Carbs: 30g, Protein: 4g

Gluten-Free Sourdough Seed and Nut Loaf

Ingredients:

- 1 cup gluten-free sourdough starter
- 2 1/2 cups gluten-free flour blend
- 1 tsp salt
- 1/4 cup mixed seeds (sunflower, pumpkin, sesame)
- 1/4 cup chopped nuts (almonds, walnuts)
- 1 tbsp honey
- 1 1/2 cups warm water
- 2 tbsp olive oil

Instructions:

1. Combine starter, flour, salt, seeds, nuts, honey, warm water, and oil in the bread machine on the dough setting.
2. Shape the dough into a loaf and place it in a greased loaf pan.
3. Bake at 375°F (190°C) for 30-35 minutes until golden brown.

- Prep Time: 20 minutes (excluding bread machine time)
- Cook Time: 30-35 minutes
- Servings: 1 loaf

Nutritional Information: (per slice) Calories: 220, Fat: 8g, Carbs: 34g, Protein: 5g

Gluten-Free Sourdough Chocolate Bread

Ingredients:

- 1 cup gluten-free sourdough starter
- 3 cups gluten-free flour blend
- 1 tsp salt
- 1/2 cup cocoa powder
- 1/2 cup sugar
- 1 cup chocolate chips
- 1 1/2 cups warm water
- 2 tbsp vegetable oil

Instructions:

1. Mix starter, flour, salt, cocoa powder, sugar, chocolate chips, warm water, and oil in the bread machine on the dough setting.
2. Once the dough is ready, shape into a loaf and place in a greased loaf pan.
3. Bake at 350°F (175°C) for 35-40 minutes until done.

- Prep Time: 15 minutes (excluding bread machine time)
- Cook Time: 35-40 minutes
- Servings: 1 loaf

Nutritional Information: (per slice) Calories: 240, Fat: 9g, Carbs: 38g, Protein: 4g

Gluten-Free Sourdough Cheese Bread

Ingredients:

- 1 cup gluten-free sourdough starter
- 2 1/2 cups gluten-free flour blend
- 1 tsp salt
- 1/2 cup grated Parmesan cheese
- 1/2 cup grated cheddar cheese
- 1 1/2 cups warm water
- 2 tbsp olive oil

Instructions:

1. In the bread machine, combine starter, flour, salt, Parmesan, cheddar, warm water, and oil using the dough setting.

2. After the cycle, shape the dough into a loaf and place in a greased loaf pan.

3. Bake at 375°F (190°C) for 30-35 minutes until golden brown.

- o   Prep Time: 15 minutes (excluding bread machine time)
- o   Cook Time: 30-35 minutes
- o   Servings: 1 loaf

Nutritional Information: (per slice) Calories: 230, Fat: 10g, Carbs: 30g, Protein: 7g

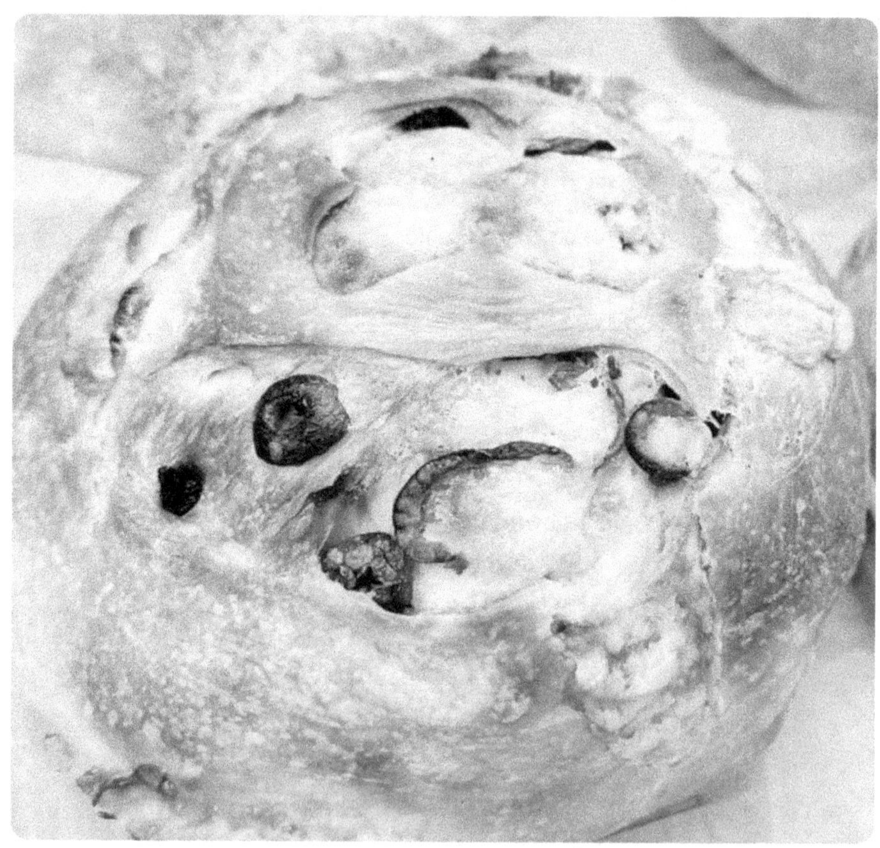

CHAPTER 7

Tips, Tricks, and Troubleshooting for Bread Machine Baking

Baking with a bread machine, especially when it comes to gluten-free sourdough, has its own set of challenges and rewards. This chapter offers valuable insights for achieving the perfect loaf directly from your bread machine, along with storage advice and solutions for common baking issues.

Achieving the Perfect Crust and Crumb in a Bread Machine

➢ Select the Right Setting: Always use the gluten-free setting if your machine has one. This setting is designed to handle the unique kneading and rising requirements of gluten-free dough.

➢ Ingredient Temperature: Ingredients should be at room temperature to ensure the yeast activates properly.

➢ Check the Dough Consistency: Gluten-free dough is generally more like a thick batter than traditional wheat dough. During the first knead cycle, open the lid and check the consistency. If it's too dry, add a tablespoon of water; if too wet, add a bit of gluten-free flour.

➢ Smooth the Top: Before the final rise, use a wet spatula to smooth the top of the dough. This helps achieve a more even crust.

Storage Advice for Bread Machine Breads

➢ Cool Before Slicing: Allow the bread to cool completely before slicing to avoid a gummy texture.

➢ Airtight Storage: Keep the bread in an airtight container to maintain freshness. Gluten-free bread tends to dry out faster.

➢ Refrigerate for Longer Freshness: If not consumed within a day, store the bread in the refrigerator.

➢ Freezing: Slice and freeze any bread you won't eat within a couple of days. You can toast slices straight from the freezer.

Troubleshooting Common Bread Machine Baking Problems

➢ Bread Not Rising: Make sure your sourdough starter is active. The temperature of the ingredients can also affect the rise. They should be at room temperature.

➢ Dense or Heavy Bread: This might be due to overmixing or not enough leavening agent. Check the freshness of your starter and the ratio of ingredients.

➢ Crumbly Bread: Gluten-free bread can be prone to crumbling due to the lack of gluten. Ensure you have enough binding agents like xanthan gum in your flour blend.

➢ Top of Bread Sinking: This can happen if there's too much liquid or yeast. Measure ingredients carefully and adjust as necessary.

➢ Uneven Crust Color: Some bread machines may bake unevenly. To mitigate this, check if your machine has a convection feature or rotate the pan halfway through baking if possible.

Baking gluten-free sourdough bread in a bread machine can be incredibly rewarding. These tips and troubleshooting ideas will help you navigate the process with greater confidence and success. Remember, each loaf is an opportunity to refine your skills and learn more about the art of gluten-free baking.

Conversion Chart

Conversion Chart for Gluten-Free Sourdough Bread Machine Cookbook

Dry Ingredients

1. Gluten-Free Flour Blend**

   - Cups to Grams: 1 cup = 120 g

- Cups to Tablespoons: 1 cup = 16 tbsp

2. Sugar

- Teaspoons to Grams: 1 tsp = 4.2 g
- Tablespoons to Grams: 1 tbsp = 12.6 g

3. Salt

- Teaspoons to Grams: 1 tsp = 5.69 g
- Tablespoons to Grams: 1 tbsp = 17.07 g

4. Baking Soda

- Teaspoons to Grams: 1 tsp = 4.6 g
- Tablespoons to Grams: 1 tbsp = 13.8 g

5. Xanthan Gum

- Teaspoons to Grams: 1 tsp = 2.6 g
- Tablespoons to Grams: 1 tbsp = 7.8 g

6. Cocoa Powder

- Cups to Grams: 1 cup = 85 g
- Tablespoons to Grams: 1 tbsp = 5.3 g

Wet Ingredients

1. Water / Milk / Milk Alternatives

- Cups to Milliliters: 1 cup = 240 ml

- Tablespoons to Milliliters: 1 tbsp = 15 ml

2. Olive Oil / Vegetable Oil / Melted Butter

- Cups to Milliliters: 1 cup = 237 ml

- Tablespoons to Milliliters: 1 tbsp = 14.79 ml

3. Honey / Maple Syrup / Molasses

- Cups to Grams: 1 cup = 340 g (approx.)

- Tablespoons to Grams: 1 tbsp = 21.25 g

Eggs

- Eggs are usually standard in size, so direct substitution is generally fine (1 egg = 1 egg).

Sourdough Starter

- The sourdough starter is typically used as is, without conversion.

Notes:

These conversions are based on standard measurements. Slight variations may occur due to differences in ingredient brands and environmental factors.

For specific ingredients like cheese, nuts, fruits, etc., it's advisable to use a kitchen scale for more accurate measurements.

Always consider the texture of the dough/batter, which might require slight adjustments in liquid or flour.

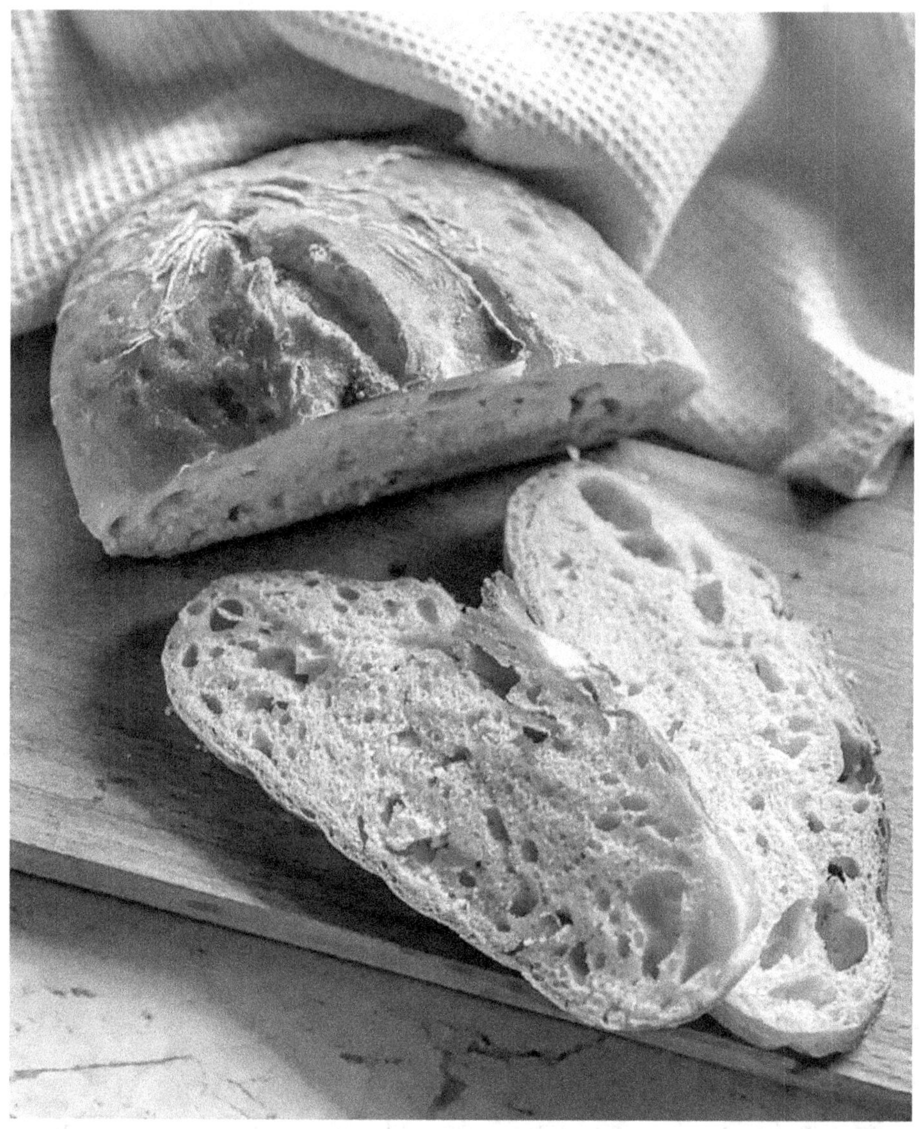

CONCLUSION

As we reach the end of our gluten-free sourdough baking journey, it's important to reflect on the path we've traveled together. From understanding the basics of gluten-free ingredients to mastering the use of your bread machine for creating sourdough delights, this book has aimed to be your steadfast companion in the kitchen.

Gluten-free baking is not just about following recipes; it's about embracing a lifestyle that prioritizes health without compromising on flavor and joy. Each chapter, each recipe in this book, was designed to bring you closer to achieving baking excellence in your own home, with the humble bread machine as your ally.

Remember, the journey of baking is filled with learning and discovery. Mistakes are merely stepping stones to success, and every loaf you bake adds to your experience. The aroma of freshly baked bread, the joy of sharing a slice with loved ones, the satisfaction of knowing you've created something wonderful with your own hands – these are the rewards that await you.

As you continue to bake, experiment, and enjoy your gluten-free sourdough creations, may you always find joy and satisfaction in the process. Keep the bread maker warm, the starter fed, and your passion for baking alive.

Acknowledgments

This book would not have been possible without the support and inspiration from a community of passionate bakers and culinary enthusiasts. A heartfelt thank you to every home baker who has fearlessly navigated the world of gluten-free sourdough, sharing their triumphs and challenges. Your experiences have been invaluable in shaping the content of this book.

Special thanks to the culinary experts and nutritionists who provided their insights on gluten-free baking, ensuring that the recipes and techniques presented are both enjoyable and health-conscious.

Gratitude is also extended to friends and family for their unwavering support and for being the ever-willing taste testers of numerous loaves. Your feedback and encouragement have been the driving force behind this endeavor.

Lastly, to you, the reader and home baker, for embarking on this journey with me. May your kitchens always be filled with the warmth of baking and your tables with the love of shared meals.

Happy baking!

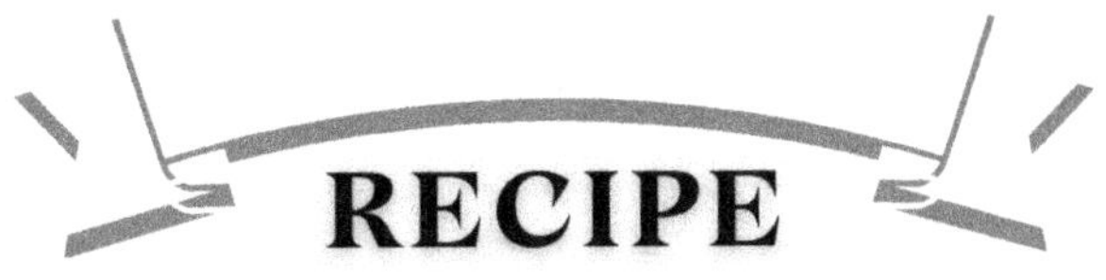

INGREDIENTS

BAKING TOOLS

SHOPPING LIST

OTHER SPICES

INSTRUCTIONS

NOTE'S

GLUTEN-FREE SOURDOUGH BREAD MACHINE COOKBOOK

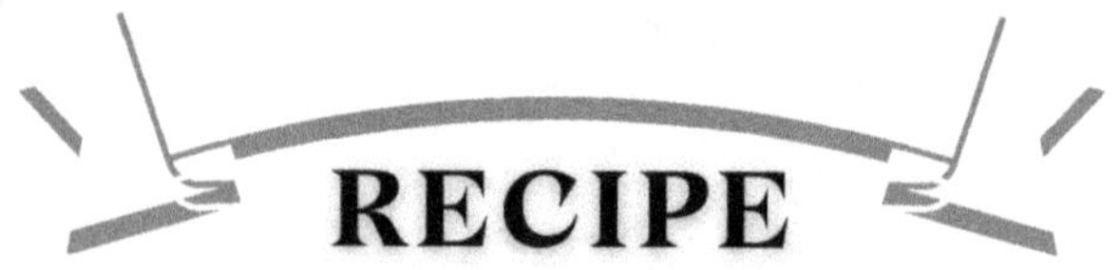

RECIPE
NAME

INGREDIENTS

BAKING TOOLS

SHOPPING LIST

OTHER SPICES

INSTRUCTIONS

NOTE'S

GLUTEN-FREE SOURDOUGH BREAD MACHINE COOKBOOK

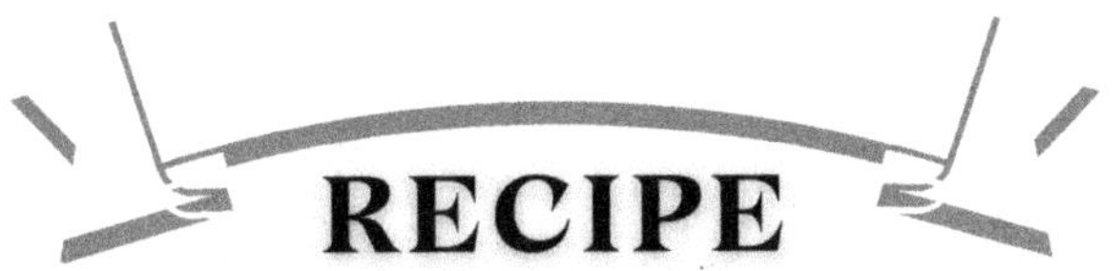

RECIPE

NAME

INGREDIENTS

BAKING TOOLS

SHOPPING LIST

OTHER SPICES

INSTRUCTIONS

NOTE'S

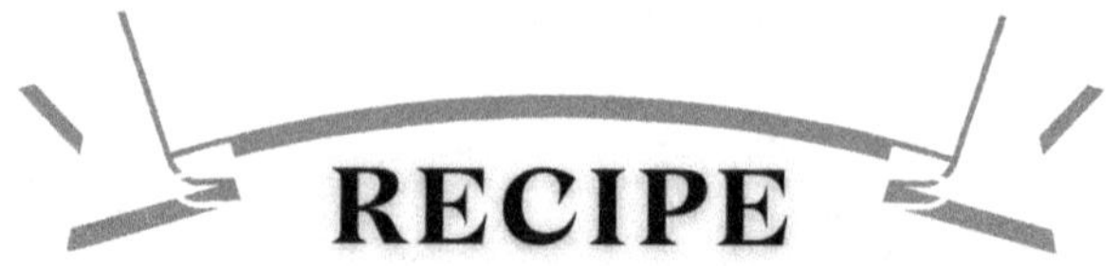

RECIPE
NAME

INGREDIENTS

BAKING TOOLS

SHOPPING LIST

OTHER SPICES

INSTRUCTIONS

NOTE'S

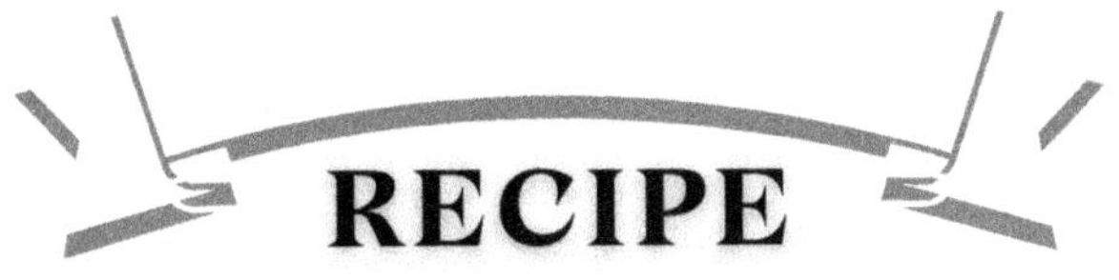

RECIPE

NAME

INGREDIENTS

BAKING TOOLS

SHOPPING LIST

OTHER SPICES

INSTRUCTIONS

NOTE'S

GLUTEN-FREE SOURDOUGH BREAD MACHINE COOKBOOK

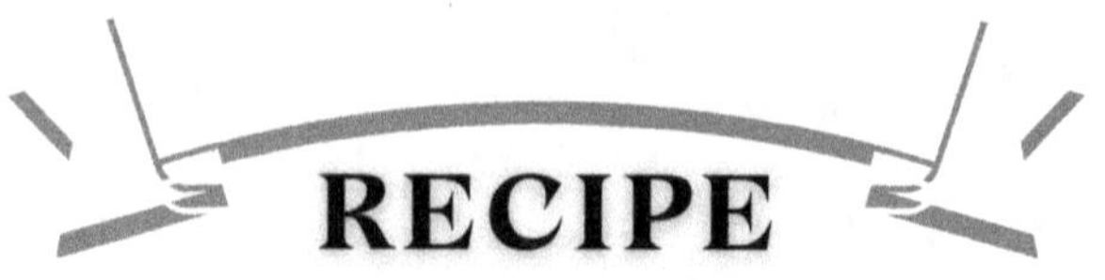

RECIPE
NAME

INGREDIENTS

BAKING TOOLS

SHOPPING LIST

OTHER SPICES

INSTRUCTIONS

NOTE'S

GLUTEN-FREE SOURDOUGH BREAD MACHINE COOKBOOK

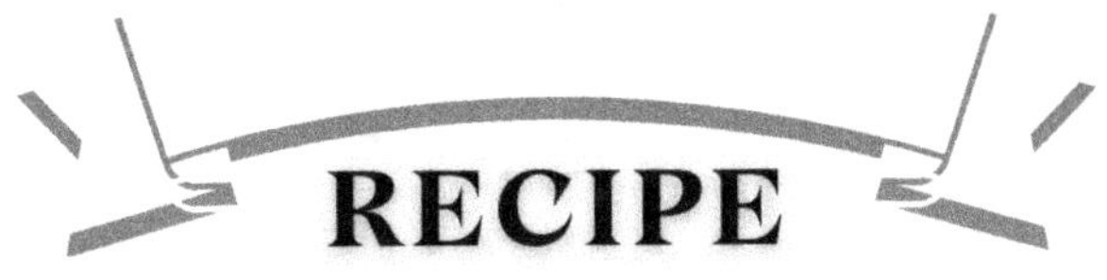

INGREDIENTS

BAKING TOOLS

SHOPPING LIST

OTHER SPICES

INSTRUCTIONS

NOTE'S

GLUTEN-FREE SOURDOUGH BREAD MACHINE COOKBOOK

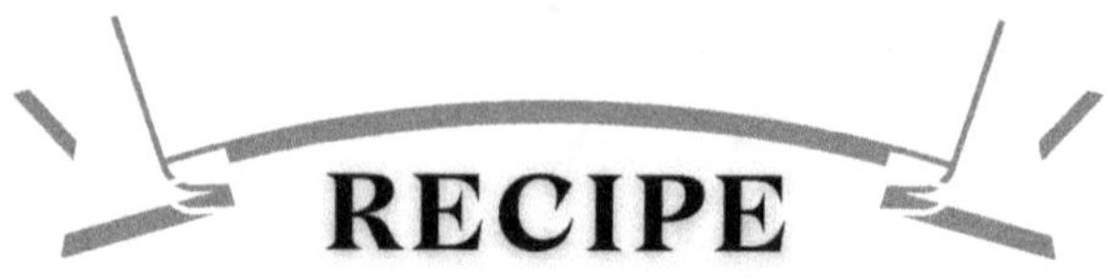

RECIPE

NAME

INGREDIENTS

BAKING TOOLS

SHOPPING LIST

OTHER SPICES

INSTRUCTIONS

NOTE'S

GLUTEN-FREE SOURDOUGH BREAD MACHINE COOKBOOK

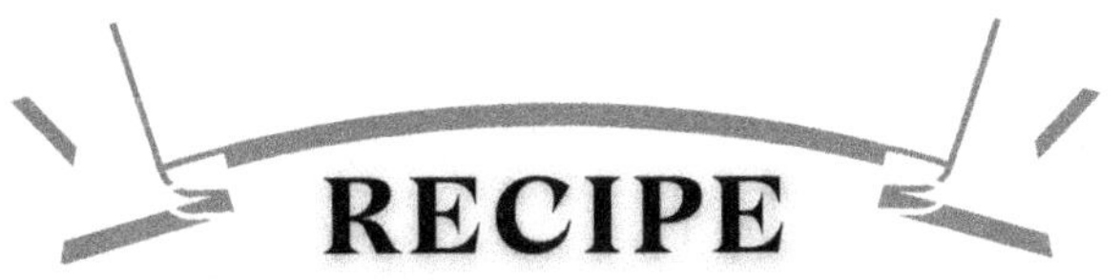

INGREDIENTS

BAKING TOOLS

SHOPPING LIST

OTHER SPICES

INSTRUCTIONS

NOTE'S

GLUTEN-FREE SOURDOUGH BREAD MACHINE COOKBOOK

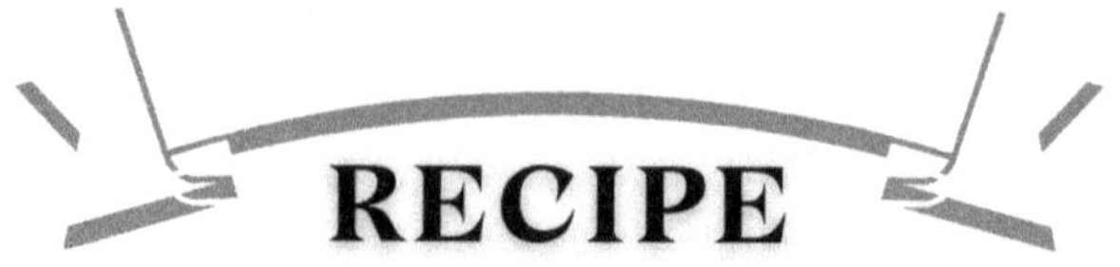

INGREDIENTS

BAKING TOOLS

SHOPPING LIST

OTHER SPICES

INSTRUCTIONS

NOTE'S

GLUTEN-FREE SOURDOUGH BREAD MACHINE COOKBOOK

INGREDIENTS

BAKING TOOLS

SHOPPING LIST

OTHER SPICES

INSTRUCTIONS

NOTE'S

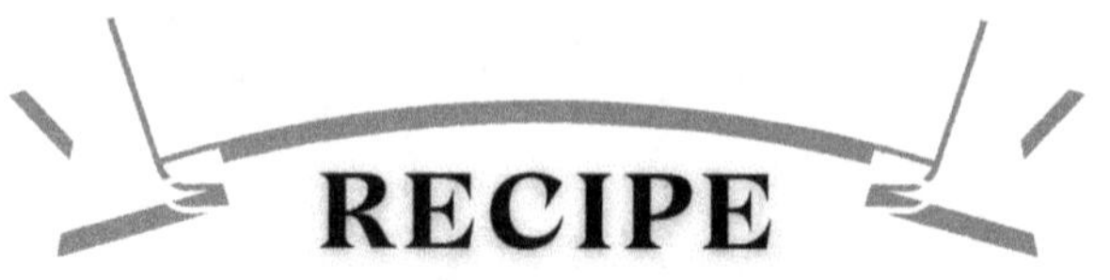

INGREDIENTS

BAKING TOOLS

SHOPPING LIST

OTHER SPICES

INSTRUCTIONS

NOTE'S

GLUTEN-FREE SOURDOUGH BREAD MACHINE COOKBOOK

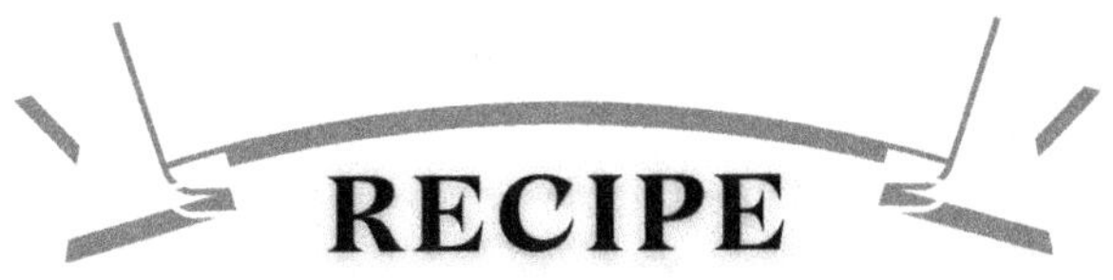

INGREDIENTS

BAKING TOOLS

SHOPPING LIST

OTHER SPICES

INSTRUCTIONS

NOTE'S

GLUTEN-FREE SOURDOUGH BREAD MACHINE COOKBOOK

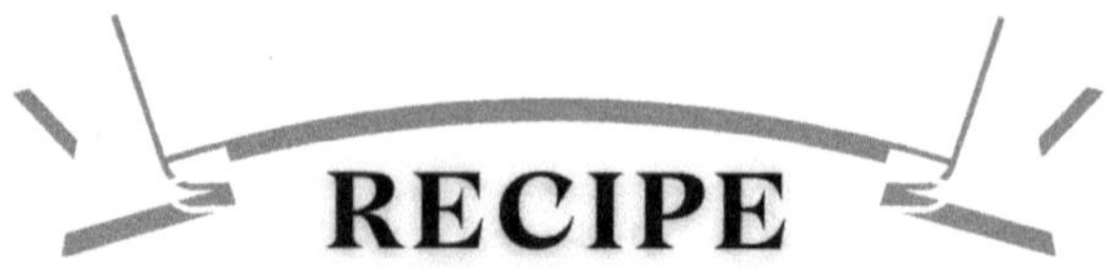

RECIPE

NAME

INGREDIENTS

BAKING TOOLS

SHOPPING LIST

OTHER SPICES

INSTRUCTIONS

NOTE'S

GLUTEN-FREE SOURDOUGH BREAD MACHINE COOKBOOK

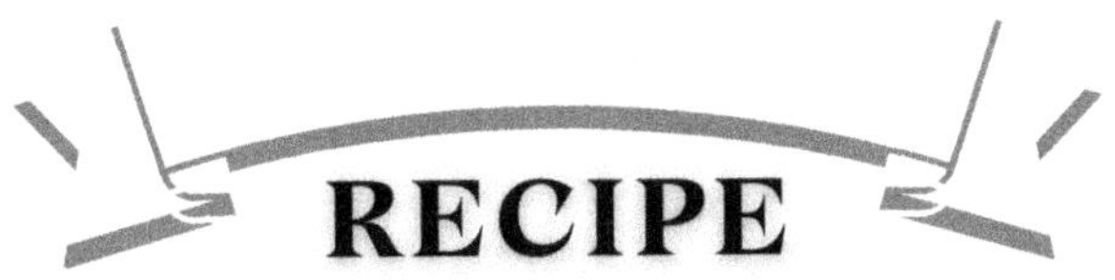

INGREDIENTS

BAKING TOOLS

SHOPPING LIST

OTHER SPICES

INSTRUCTIONS

NOTE'S

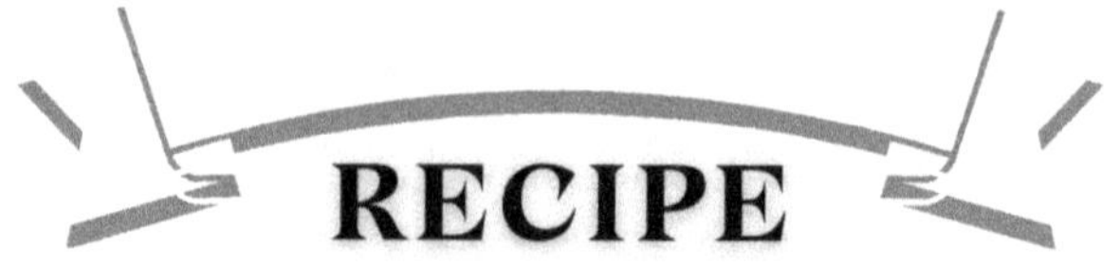

RECIPE
NAME

INGREDIENTS

BAKING TOOLS

SHOPPING LIST

OTHER SPICES

INSTRUCTIONS

NOTE'S

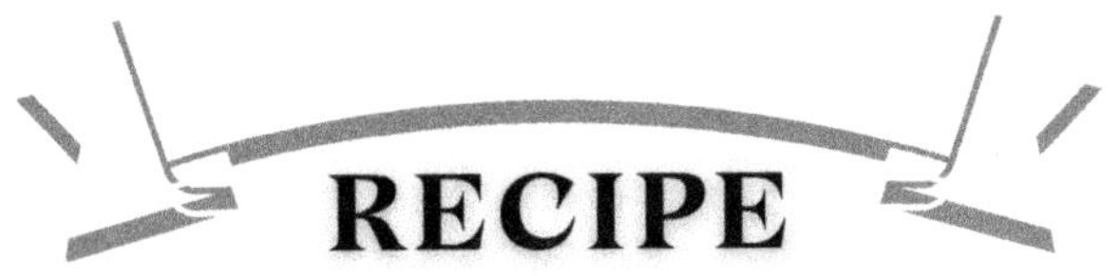

RECIPE
NAME

INGREDIENTS

BAKING TOOLS

SHOPPING LIST

OTHER SPICES

INSTRUCTIONS

NOTE'S

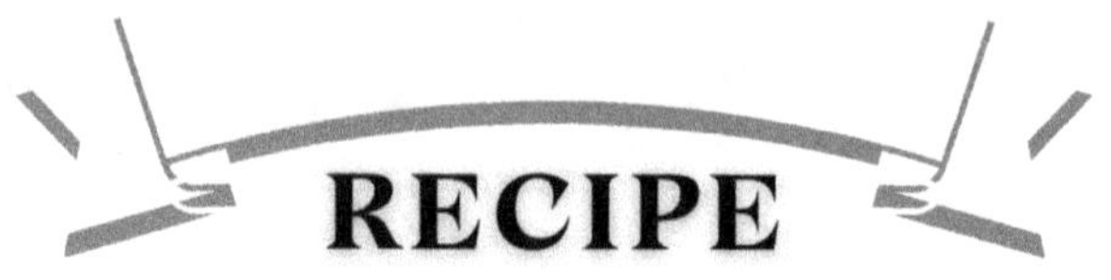

RECIPE

NAME

INGREDIENTS

BAKING TOOLS

SHOPPING LIST

OTHER SPICES

INSTRUCTIONS

NOTE'S

GLUTEN-FREE SOURDOUGH BREAD MACHINE COOKBOOK

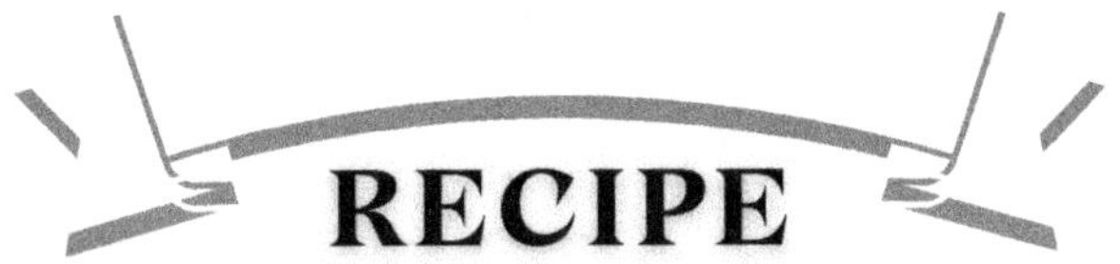

RECIPE
NAME

INGREDIENTS

BAKING TOOLS

SHOPPING LIST

OTHER SPICES

INSTRUCTIONS

NOTE'S

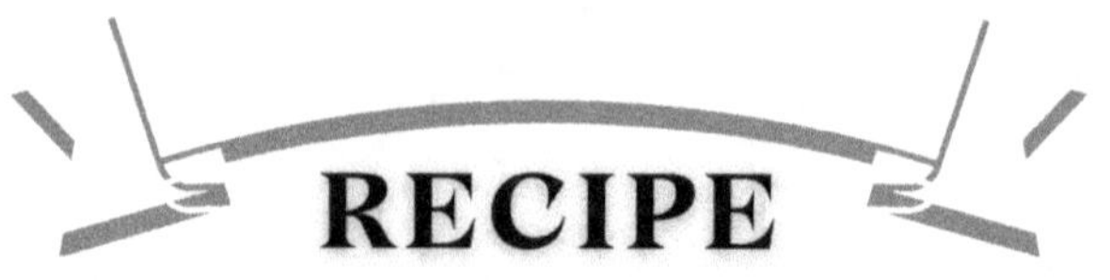

RECIPE
NAME

INGREDIENTS

BAKING TOOLS

SHOPPING LIST

OTHER SPICES

INSTRUCTIONS

NOTE'S